Doing Child and Adolescent Psychotherapy

Doing Child and Adolescent Psychotherapy

Adapting Psychodynamic Treatment to Contemporary Practice

Second Edition

Richard Bromfield, Ph.D.

John Wiley & Sons, Inc.

Published by John Wiley & Sons, Inc., Hoboken, New Jersey.
Published simultaneously in Canada.

Wiley Bicentennial Logo: Richard J. Pacifico

For general information on our other products and services please contact our Customer Care
Department within the United States at (800) 762–2974, outside the United States at (317)
572–3993 or fax (317) 572–4002.

Wiley also publishes its books in a variety of electronic formats. Some content that appears in
print may not be available in electronic books. For more information about Wiley products, visit
our web site at www.wiley.com.

Library of Congress Cataloging-in-Publication Data:
Bromfield, Richard.
    Doing child and adolescent psychotherapy : adapting psychodynamic treatment to
contemporary practice, second edition / Richard Bromfield.
        p. ; cm.
    Includes bibliographical references and indexes.
    ISBN 978–0–470–12181–8 (cloth : alk. paper)
    1. Child psychotherapy.   2. Adolescent psychotherapy.   3. Psychodynamic
psychotherapy.   4. Play therapy.   I. Title.
    [DNLM: 1. Psychotherapy—methods.   2. Adolescent.   3. Child. WS 350.2 B868d 2007]
    RJ504.B753 2007
    618.92'8914—dc22
                                                                                2007002738

Printed in the United States of America.

10 9 8 7 6 5 4 3 2 1

For Margo, friend and mentor

Contents

vii

What's New to the Second Edition

Almost 10 years ago I wrote a guide to child therapy. I worked hard, then, to make the book relevant, timely, and thorough. But a lot has happened over the past decade. The economics of mental health, a euphemism for managed care and insurance companies, have grown from supporters of what we do to dictators of it. Even as we meet with our young patients in the privacy of our offices, we feel those bureaucratic beasts breathing down our necks. If, just as Watergate's Deep Throat advised, we "follow the money," we see the profound influence that these entities have had on the important work we do. Hospital beds and inpatient settings are disappearing. Every day, child therapists are asked to do more with fewer resources in less time. Paperwork, legal matters, and compliance with state and federal regulations have, like greedy little Pacmen, rushed in ahead of patients to gobble up clinicians' time.

But the shrinking dollar for child treatment has done even more than stress child therapy and its providers. Through the subtle powers of the mental health market, our field has started to join rather than fight. Short-term models of therapy and evidence-based interventions have ascended. Under the strain of financial realities, clinicians find it harder to stick to what they believe or are downright prevented from doing so. However precious their mission, child therapists work for a living just like everyone else. To use a weak analogy, a house might need scraping, a primer, and two final coats. If we are going to be paid for only one final coat, how many of us can afford to do it properly? The discrepancy between ideal practice and what really exists has expanded into a Great Divide.

Yet it would be too easy to dismiss these new treatments and their research as nothing more than quick and dirty ways to save a buck or, a bit more generously, as means to survive in today's more competitive environment. While the pursuit of cheaper and quicker treatment methods might be driven by other than benevolent forces, the men and women who are studying those treatments genuinely want to help children faster and more effectively. There is no virtue in getting better slowly. Anything that alleviates children's pain and promotes their growth in less time is to be honored and adopted.

Real differences exist, and we won't shy away from them. We live in a new world order, however, one that we have to and should reckon with. This new and second edition of *Doing Child and Adolescent Therapy* will take up this challenge—holding on to all we know about the value of relationships, personal meanings, and inner worlds to children, their difficulties, and their recoveries—while heeding what we are learning about other ways to help them and their families. At times, we will change our minds, sometimes integrating and accommodating. At other times, we'll acknowledge the debatable truths of both sides. And then, many times, we'll stay put, not stubbornly or out of ignorance but for what we judge to be good reason.

To be a contemporary guide to child therapy, my book will need to do more, and it will. Its sturdy spine, centered around the therapist–child relationship, will follow a timely trajectory that spans from the initial referral call, through early assessment through the middle substance of therapy on to termination. The first third of the book, *The Essentials,* will address how we begin a treatment, how it works, the mechanics of therapeutic powers and need for limits, and the techniques of therapeutic talk and query. The middle third, *Techniques and Tools,* in pragmatic and lively terms will detail the use of puppet play, toys, games, and art in child therapy, paying special attention to the ways we balance play *and talk*. Here, we'll also deal with the exceptions of therapy, such as gift giving, disclosing, and bending the framework. Despite its lazy title, the final section, *The Rest*, ambitiously tackles parent guidance, family work, reluctant patients, crisis, medication, diversity and cultural dynamics, managed care and evidence-based treatment, and concluding a therapy—a miscellany critical to child therapy.

I've aspired to address all that matters, writing in prose that is clear and engaging, that shows as much as tells, and that conveys the real experience that child therapists will immediately recognize. In the end, only you will judge the relevance of this book to your precious work as a child therapist. I hope it proves itself worth your time.

Preface to the First Edition

Wᵉ child therapists need no convincing of the seriousness and arduousness of our mission. In our most splendid moments, we see our young patients heal and go forth on solid ground toward happier and more satisfying lives. At other and more usual times, we help children and their parents get through another day or week with less mishap and destruction or, perhaps, leave our offices with a little less pain and suffering than when they came. And sadly, there are the darkest times, when our best efforts do not help at all.

Our purpose is not, as some observers think, simply to be a friend or confidant to the child. That would be easy. As I've written elsewhere (Bromfield, 1992, p. 6), children's playing in therapy is much more than mere "fun or pretend-to-be-taken seriously." What we do is complex, wearing, slow, and uncertain in its progress and outcome. And much of what we do we do alone—without help, confirmation, or encouragement, often against the odds or under disapproving eyes. Done properly, being a child therapist is hard and noble work.

This book is dedicated to that worthy and challenging purpose. With vivid clinical material and personal candor, the theoretical essence and practical essentials of doing child and adolescent psychotherapy are laid out, from the referral call to the last good-bye, capturing the intricacies and subtleties of children and their therapies in their biggest and smallest ways—and everywhere in between. Whatever aspect of therapy is discussed, our eyes and ears are aimed toward what is transpiring in the child, in the therapist, and in the space they share. And whatever the clinical situation being examined, a slow and steady focus on the building and meaning of relationships—between child and family, child and world, child and therapist, inner and outer experience—ever reigns supreme in these pages. The belief that the therapist's most powerful, if not sole, therapeutic tool is himself pervades every nook and cranny of the book and serves as its foundation.

I hope this intimate and pragmatic guide to child psychotherapy renews, fortifies, and enriches the important work you, as child therapist, pursue every moment of every clinical hour.

—RB, 1997

Acknowledgments

How does one thank the near-countless colleagues, supervisors, supervisees, and patients who have taught me hour by hour since I first walked in, on wobbly knees, to meet my first child in therapy? I hope those who have taught me best can see and hear themselves in these pages. Gratitude goes to Patricia Rossi, my editor at Wiley, who from a small correspondence we had years ago held on to her belief in a readable book to integrate psychodynamic child therapy with the realities and resources of modern health care. And a special thanks go to Dr. Gene Beresin, whose review of this book's first edition, a decade ago, served as a compass for its dramatic changes, revision, and enrichment.

To the Reader

As I wrote previously, "I use *children* to mean children and adolescents of all ages. If I need to define a child or group more narrowly, I use other terms, such as infant, toddler, adolescent, or first-grader. I refer to those I see in therapy as *patients* (though I appreciate the sentiments of those preferring the term *clients*). When speaking about children or therapists in general, I randomly alternate male and female pronouns to avoid the intolerable monotony of he and she, her or him" (Bromfield, 1992, p. 9).

Doing Child and Adolescent Psychotherapy

Part I

The Essentials

1

Easy Does It: Beginning Therapy

Beginnings are important, arguably critical. A small misstep can detour us unnecessarily; a large enough one can wholly derail the journey. At the very least, the first steps, the ones from which all other steps follow, form the foundation on which a therapy and the essential relationship within are built.

We begin with the parents. They are the ones who usually choose, arrange, and pay for a child's psychotherapy. Consider the challenge facing the mothers and fathers who call us. In a handful of minutes, they try their best to present an enormously complicated, painful, and often embarrassing situation to a complete stranger who purports to be some kind of expert on matters of children and families. As former students, we know the intellectual demand of case formulation. Imagine adding the heavy measure of worry, self-blame, and hopelessness that parents feel.[1]

Whatever parents' issues, we try to listen patiently. If we're rushed, we say so and offer a better time in the near future to talk. Sensitized to the difficulty of their call, we try to help parents tell their story—asking helpful questions of the timid, slowing the speedy, organizing the rambling. We do so not only to foster a connection but also to see what the problem is and whether it is one that we can help solve.

A few more moments on the phone can convince us that we are not the appropriate clinician and might inform our making an effective referral elsewhere. Or they can help us to distinguish true crises from entitled demands or reveal the basic motive for the call (e.g., seeking not therapy for the child but evidence to battle for custody). Our time is well spent on the first call and is in everyone's best interest. It preserves our hours to do treatment. It saves the patient's time and money, and, by helping get the child to the right help and person, it can prevent the emotional toll of prematurely investing in the wrong therapist.

When sensing a mismatch, we gently—so as to minimize any feelings of rejection—describe how children, particularly adolescents, tend to connect most with the therapist they see first. Meeting with us, we further explain, could obstruct connecting with a second therapist. For many parents and children, meeting a therapist and sharing their stories is both draining and bonding. It is almost always best to save the powerful early meetings for the therapist of final destination (though sometimes clinical conditions or the restraints of health care systems require patients to see a series of practitioners on the way to their eventual clinician).

While we assess matters, so do parents. In many instances, they shop for a therapist even as we speak. What do parents look for? All sorts of things. Facts, such as what we do, what we charge, what kinds of insurance we accept, whether we have openings, where the office is. Do we listen and seem to care? Do we sound kindly and patient?

Many parents have begun to form impressions of us even before hearing our voices. If we've come highly recommended, there may be halos around our heads. While inflated views of what we can do make for easier and enthusiastic beginnings, they can just as often backfire, leading to disappointment and impatience, even premature endings, when our work does not produce big enough or fast enough results.

Conversely—and more commonly in today's busy and tight marketplace—parents consult us because of insurance plan constraints or matters of distance and scheduling. To one disgruntled mother who saw me as her distant second choice, I said, "You've mentioned several times having to stick to a list of providers." Putting such dissatisfaction on the table helped her to speak her mind concerning her ultimate doubt as to whether any therapist could help. Sharing this thought with me gave her a bit more confidence in the process and led to her giving me a fair chance to prove myself with her and her daughter.

I see the purpose of the initial call as deciding whether future contact with me is likely to benefit the child. If it makes sense that we go no further, I aspire to give parents a good experience with me as representative of the mental health profession so that they will persist in their quest for help. And when we do agree to meet in person, this call has gotten us off on surer footing, the work well begun.

FIRST MEETINGS

With younger children, I typically offer parents the option of meeting with me first without their child. This provides an opportunity for the parents to speak freely and check me out. I suggest that parents of elementary school children accompany their child. In contrast, I urge parents to let their teenage children come to the beginning hour by themselves, explaining that doing so counters the common adolescent tendency to mistrust and reject the therapist as another arm of parental authority. I bend, however, to comply with parents' good reasons for other arrangements (e.g., a ninth-grade girl who fears going anywhere without her mother or including a very young sibling who can't be left alone in the waiting room). Regardless of the child's age, in the course of the initial meetings I try to meet with both child and parents, alone and together. This early negotiating, structuring, and educating concerning who should come begins to show parents how therapy will work and proceed.

Making our patients feel safe—the absolute first requisite to any worthwhile course of therapy—begins in the earliest moments. Do we take a minute to greet everyone who has come with the child? Are we kindly? Do we smile sincerely? Do we look the child and his mother in the eye? Or do we appear to be just doing a job, grudgingly serving the next customer? Do we ask how they're doing, then turn away and head into the office before they've answered? Giving a disorganized mother a few minutes to gather her children and their belongings may accomplish more than rushing her into the office. By themselves insufficient to ensure good treatment, these civilities—done in good measure, neither to feign sympathy nor to manipulate—convey a sense of us as real persons and help our patients make the transition to the world of therapy they're about to enter.

When we go out to meet new child patients, some zip past us like Speedy Gonzalez, rifling through our toy boxes or our desks before we've said hello. A majority of them follow the lead of their parents who, in turn, follow ours. Others dally, coming at a snail's pace out of fear or to show who's boss.

Sure that I, at this point, am sure of little, I tend to stay out of the line of fire. I let parents and child struggle their way into the office, reminding myself that they somehow manage their lives when I am not around. I do not force anyone to come in, for that is the quickest way to nowhere. My threats or tugs may get a reluctant child inside today, but there's a good chance he won't return tomorrow. And even if the child returns, she will see me as someone to be mistrusted, someone who has little respect for what she wants and does. Frustrating as it is, we generally can't hurry what must come in its own time.

I can't recall one instance when I've denied a child's wish to come in with or without someone. Soon after we settle in, however, I turn our attention to the reasons for the demand, leading to a readjusting of who should and shouldn't be there. While I never force a child to separate from a parent, I do note the desperate nature of her fear, a fear that will quickly take center stage in her therapy.

When parents can't get a child to even come to the waiting room, I spend my time consulting with them, helping them to better understand and manage their child. Anything but a waste, such sessions prove to be at least as valuable as if the child had come (which usually happens the following week).

Once in the office, I say hello again. Children seem to appreciate this and sense that, under their parents' and my watchful eyes, they hadn't had a good chance to meet me. After a minute of quiet, an awful lot of children will spontaneously comment on what happened in the waiting room—the confusion, the nagging, the sibling riot—shedding light on their thinking and family dynamics. My simple interest in these observations goes further than any proclamations I might make to show my accepting attitude. The actual words, "You can say anything you want in here," however exuberantly stated, have in themselves convinced very few children to spill the beans.

For the first minutes of our hour, I allow children to do as they wish. Some children calmly survey the place before taking aim at a particular object or toy. Some go right to my desk and begin drawing or ask if they may. Some come close; some stay as far away as they can. Nontherapists may be surprised to learn that many children sit in the chair opposite mine and begin talking of their troubles or wait for me to ask about them.

By this time, children tend to take notice of the office. Is it a place for children? This, perhaps, is the first question our child patients try to answer for themselves. Children from almost any background and class seem to prefer comfortable, cozy, and unpretentious. They prefer offices that look more like living rooms than hospital suites. Children tend to pick cluttered over immaculate, assuming that they will not be expected to be as neat in their play (and maybe even in their thoughts). And as we all know, a good selection of toys, building and drawing materials, and the like can be the quickest route to making children feel welcome (though, to be sure, it takes a lot more than cool stuff to earn their confidence).

Children will look around in an attempt to learn about the therapist. Fine furniture and original oil paintings will certainly give a different impression than ripped posters put out by the dairy council or drug companies. Happy childish pictures of sleeping bunnies and dogs dressed in people's clothes may entertain but give a much different impression than more sedate and ambiguous pictures of roads winding into the woods or a lone bird flying into a muted seascape. Too many diplomas may impress one child, make a second feel inferior, and lead a third to perceptively wonder about the therapist's insecurity. Children begin to read into what they see, but most of the time will keep it to themselves in the first hour, over time testing their hypotheses against the real thing, the therapist.

Of course, many child therapists don't have their own offices. They, as students or as practitioners in a crowded clinic, use whatever room is available, however poorly kept or offensively decorated. Other therapists do their work on the road, hauling a bag of toys to schools and shelters. These therapists know best what the rest of us learn soon enough, that over the long haul it is our psychological presence, not our furnishings or things, that most matter to patients.

To learn and be able to help all we can, we need children and their parents to talk as openly as possible. To talk they must be comfortable. How do we accomplish that?

We might actively seduce them, by permitting them to sit on the win-dowsills, offering soda and chips, whatever the hour. We might alleviate the slightest hint of tension, theirs or ours, by laughing robustly at things that do not strike us as funny or that are unusually perverted. Likewise, we can compliment their parents' choice of clothes or disclose that we, too, have children who wet their beds or disobey us. But these methods carry risk. Children and parents may get the wrong idea of what we do, thinking that we are there to appease them rather than to help them confront their demons and troubles.

Giving good ear is the earliest and most powerful method we have to engage parents and children. By *good ear,* I mean listening that is atten-tive and caring, listening that truly wants to hear what is being said, not that wants mostly to get another question and interview out of the way. While patients' words inevitably evoke thoughts and feelings in us, we cannot really listen while planning our next question. Some of us nod and others "ahem" in understanding. But it is the substance of our listen-ing that underlies these signs, the where and how it leads us, that shows parents and children that we are there and interested.

We may have a million questions; we ask a limited number. We ask them slowly. No one likes a third degree, even those who deserve inter-rogation. Too many questions can shut down the most open and coop-erative of us. A handful of open-ended questions answered fully and with ample reflection and interaction will, on the average, inform us more than a lengthy laundry list of items to be asked and responded to Dragnet style.

We go cautiously and remind ourselves that not every piece of infor-mation is an invitation for further probing. Patients will often tell more than they wish to and more than they are comfortable with. Learning who our patients are takes time and cannot be jammed into one, two, or even three sessions (even if mandated so by a health care insurer).

Knowing also means knowing when we don't know. On hearing of a dead grandfather, I've made the mistake of inferring sadness and regret, later learning from an embarrassed teenager that, in fact, she was glad that "that son of a bitch" had died, a pillar of his community who'd abused his daughter, my patient's mother. I don't assume to know what anything means to another person I'm just meeting. "Why," I'll ask a parent, "do you think Ben (a seventh grader) is so worried about getting into college now?" Or, "Why, of all the different issues you've raised, are you most upset about Joan's not being more popular?" "What's making you cry?" I'll softly ask a child who weeps. And when she says, "I don't know," I may gently wonder aloud whether she is sure that she really doesn't. Those I ask are often surprised that I question matters or behaviors that tend to be taken at face value. Their varied and unexpected answers confirm the wisdom of my inquiring.

Although we may not like what we are told, our job is neither to judge nor to criticize. We can take for granted that our parents and child patients have already gotten a lifetime's worth of judgment and to little avail. Experiencing our respect for their lifestyle, they—the ones who sought us—frequently will reveal on their own what they think to be amiss or at fault. By *respect*, I mean appreciation of the meaning and value that certain life decisions have had for others. I mean neither enthusiastic praise nor tacit endorsement, for it is quite possible that sooner or later I will help parents see why some of their choices have been harmful or deterring to their child—and maybe to themselves. Similarly, we must respect the love that a child has for her parents and families, however abusive or mistreating. To neglect or unilaterally dismiss that love or relationship is to neglect the child.

Our neutrality toward interpersonal conflicts as well as those within the child centers our compass so we can position ourselves to best see all that transpires. I am repulsed, for instance, when a young boy describes torturing animals. But I know that my moral censure will only send this child away to hurt more animals—and perhaps people, including himself. Listening to the gory details and slowly discovering the hurts and injuries that lead to his need for cruel power are, relatively speaking, the surest key to helping him stop his wayward sadism.

Similarly, when I observe a boy and his father wrestle, I do not take sides. My hunches about who is most right almost always prove to be wrong in the long run. Besides, it really does take two to tango, even when the two are parent and child. Our clear role is to aid both parties to assume responsibility for their contribution, whether 5 percent or 95.

Fearing criticism and not knowing what to expect, parents and their children may be quite nervous when they come to meet us. Often, just seeing that we are regular people and that our offices have chairs and lamps and wallpaper—not medical machinery or rubber pads—can moderate that anxiety. Managing the tension that remains or that is made anew in response to our interviewing is another major way to foster comfort.

We don't want our patients to feel too stressed to speak and think or so ill at ease with the process that they abandon therapy before it begins. Nor do we want patients to feel so relaxed they lose the impetus to do the work that therapy requires. Overly successful attempts to reduce patients' stress can make for easier sessions but can risk letting parents and children leave feeling as alone with their problems as when they came.

How do we concretely manage tension? We watch and observe patients' reactions to the interview setting and our comments. Unless we know how to see anxiety, we can do little to handle it. In some children, it's easy to see. They visibly shake and sweat, squirm in their seats, put bracelets on and take them off, or pick their noses. Some talk at the speed of light, compulsively interrupt us and themselves, and overflow with a cascade of worry.

Tension can be harder to detect in others. It can hide behind seemingly self-composed personas that are more guarded than confident. Or it can be the motive pushing more aggressive parents to confront us about our credentials or skills before we, so they fear, can attack them first. Likewise, children who seem to want little to do with us may be revealing, not so much an active rejection of us, but a morbid fear of people.

We seldom remark directly on a nervous habit for that can make patients feel criticized and self-conscious and take away an outlet for their tension. But noting the enormity of their anxiety—"You're holding so much worry"—in words that connote the painful burden of being a worrier can help. Overtly nervous children respond to calm and steadiness and even humor concerning their plight. We do not falsely reassure, telling them that they or their loved ones will never die, for that does not reassure and mostly makes us seem like fools.

We go slowly with patients whose anxiety is withdrawn or disguised. When children physically step back, we do not step forward or even lean forward. Their retreat is for good and deep reason. We do not force eye contact. Or should a child be fortressed in his winter coat, we do not rush to invite him to take it off. We assume he feels better with his coat on. When children psychically withdraw, we honor that too, letting their neglect of our questions go for now.

As therapists, our flexible use of structure and freedom helps to create a sense of safety. I find that a majority of patients, children and parents, do best with a relatively open-ended atmosphere that, while mindful of the information I need to know, follows their lead. This is not as true for others. The freedom to do or say as they wish can immobilize some anxious and inhibited patients. They prefer guidance as to where to sit, what to talk about, how to play. Rambunctious and impulsive patients are bolstered by greater structure and sharp limits.

Depressive children and parents may have other requisites for comfort and safety. They need therapists who can tolerate great sadness and despair, even this early in the relationship. The glib cheer of a Pollyanna will leave them untouched and awash. They need therapists who take their pain and hopelessness seriously without falling prey to their gloomy outlook. Such patients require enough silence in the hour for their hurts and passivity to surface.

Narcissistic children and parents have especially strong needs not to feel flawed or lacking. Just coming to see a therapist can feel like a frontal assault to the esteem of narcissistically fragile people. We take great care to note the courage—and for parents the great love, too—implicit in their coming for help. We tiptoe, not out of fear but to prevent sudden and disruptive deflating of a self-image that, however large, is quite shaky. When they ask unusual or abundant questions about our qualifications, we answer straightforwardly and nondefensively. We hold these children and parents with great care lest they drop, break, and flee the shame of therapy.

And then there are the angry parents and children who have come with great ambivalence or against their will, under the pressure of a spouse, school, or court. Sometimes simply acknowledging and accepting their reluctant presence defuses the anger and allows the interview to proceed smoothly. Others may be comforted and put into a manageable place by our clear stance that we will not be mistreated.

Both parents and children appreciate our sincere interest in their story, in knowing why they have come. "The school says that Joey has ADD. But what do *you* think?" I ask a parent, my question paying homage to the importance of *their* opinion of *their* child and suggesting that they will be expected to participate. From child to mother to father I go, asking each for his or her version, inviting each to critique or confirm the others' view, trying to find the discrepancies and announce the truths that always lie in the middle. "Joey, you're telling me that you can get so wild it scares you. And your parents are telling me that they've been getting on your back, sometimes even being mean, because they don't know what to do when you get that wild. Is that something you all would like help with?" Stated matter-of-factly and in their own terms, parents and child appreciate clear summaries of the reasons they've come.

Our valuing free expression will show itself early and clearly. Unlike what occurs with many other authorities in their lives, children are pleasantly surprised and sometimes bemused to see that they can say whatever they like, however they like. Whether it's about sex, aggression, greed, or silliness, they discover that it's okay in here. They can put down their teachers, their parents, and even me without being punished or retaliated against. They soon see that our only revenge is to gently wonder what experiences might account for their feelings and opinions.

When a young girl stammers to tell her side of the story to a bullying parent, I hold my finger to my lips, shushing the parent to let the child speak. I am no less protective of a devoted mother whose teenage and somewhat abusing son cuts her off at every word. My interruptions are meant not to ridicule or control but to facilitate talking. Both parents and children start to learn what therapy and I am about.

Although therapists have an agenda, meaning certain things we want to know, we are bound to it loosely. We follow the lead of the children and parents, the ones who live their lives firsthand. Their consciouses and unconsciouses know the quickest shortcuts as well as the most telling detours around the issues and pains that bring them here. Our overactivity—too many questions, too many what-abouts, too many changed subjects—will likely distract us and our patients from the matters at hand and in their hearts.

These generic ways of being with children and their parents in the first meetings give them something immediate and tangible to know about us and therapy, begin to forge a sense of trust and relationship, and promote our gathering the information we need to more formally plan and offer treatment.[2]

NOTES

1. Frederick Allen (1964) makes clear that, whatever the circumstances, parents' bringing their child for help is a "first step of prime importance for them" (p. 101). Allen aptly stresses the unique and intense experience that the first meeting evokes for both children and their parents. His enlightening

chapter can be found in *Child Psychotherapy*, a book edited by Mary Haworth. Its list of contributing authors—Erik Erikson, Virginia Axline, Eveoleen Rexford, Clark Moustakas, Melanie Klein, Haim Ginott, Jessie Taft, Anna Freud, Selma Fraiberg, and so on—reads like a Who's Who of child psychotherapy. The rich, useful, and brief pieces in Haworth's compilation remain highly relevant to today's therapists. They also give a good sense of the history and state of the field in the 1960s.

2. Students and trainees will especially appreciate the chapter by Shapiro, Friedberg, and Bardenstein (2006) on therapy fundamentals. They offer valuable and concrete suggestions on ways to meet and talk with the child and parents. See also Anna Freud's discussion on introducing treatment to the child (Sandler, Kennedy, & Tyson, 1980, pp. 153–157) and Reisman's (1973) chapter "Meeting the Child" (pp. 121–156).

2

Can I Help You? Evaluating the Child and Offering Treatment

Parents want to feel safe and understood, and they want their children to feel the same. But the prime reason they are here is that they want us to stop their child's problem behaviors, relieve her distressing symptoms, and help her cope with difficult life circumstances.

Before we can help, we need to assess the child to determine whether therapy makes sense and, if so, whether we are the clinicians most suited to provide it. To this end, the early meetings are as evaluative as they are therapeutic.

GETTING TO KNOW THE CHILD

Almost too obvious to mention, the first piece of information we collect is the parents' stated reason for coming. These leading complaints can describe what is most pressing to the parents or at least what they feel most comfortable sharing at this early stage. "Gwen is failing in school."

"Alejandro's been getting stomachaches and not wanting to leave the house." "Billy just seems too angry for a third grader. Everything throws him into a rage."

For the boy whose parents mention rage, I am particularly watchful for signs of anger or undue frustration. If they are not apparent, I wonder why he doesn't show them to me. Is he overly polite or submissive to me, or does his quickness to flare show itself when he rejoins his parents at the hour's end? Perhaps he is not hot-tempered at all but has a mother who cannot tolerate conflict and who herself is furious much of the time over being abandoned by her husband. Whatever other symptoms and issues eventually show up, however more complex, the parents' original reasons for referral serve to organize our interviewing and formulating.

When we first meet, we are equally interested in hearing what the child thinks are the reasons for his seeing a therapist. Although many children reflexively answer that they don't know, most cannot help but give their side, often interrupting their parents' versions. Even young children can sometimes describe something about why they are here. Of the ones who can't, a good number, with our help, can confirm or negate what we or their parents suggest. Children will frequently cite accurately their bad behaviors and others' disapproval as the main factors for their parents bringing them, filling in the acts and symptoms they themselves are bothered by only if given the time, space, and caring encouragement to do so.

Drawing on our experience with child patients and children we have known out of the office, we try to put the parents' and children's perspective into (our) perspective. Are their concerns excessive, like those of one father who saw impending catastrophe in his high school daughter's first C? (His unrealistic standards, not her grade, became the focus of our work.) Or are these concerns out of whack in the other direction? "We know he's been using acid lately, but all the kids are, aren't they?"

The timeliness of the referral provides further understanding. "At least four years," one mother replied to my query as to how long her son had been doing things to hurt himself. "But until this past fall he'd just pull out his hair and scratch himself till he bled." In several cases, I've recalled to myself that the parents seeing me today had called me one, two, or many years ago and then postponed their decision for therapy; some had even made appointments they never kept. Are they frightened, procrastinating, denying parents, I wonder? Or are they ambivalent about getting their child help or having a clinician meddle in their affairs?

Are the parents interested in the child's perceptions? Most parents who bring their children are. But some parents, often those who were pushed here by schools or other agencies, want us to know only the ways in which their children do bad and disrupt their (the parents') lives. Such parents grow impatient with us when we ask their little girl what she thinks and where she hurts. They may read our interest as weak and pandering to a child they have come to see as controlling and not to be trusted.

When the main complaint is a specific behavior, we ask concrete questions. When, why, and how much? "Does he mouth off everywhere or just at home or maybe just with you?" Whatever the problem, be it an eating disturbance or school suspension, we want details. "Tell me," I ask parents and children who fight too much, "when's the last time you battled? What happened? How did it start? How did it end? Was it upsetting, uninvolving or . . ."—yes, families will confirm with embarrassed smiles—". . . fun?" Our pursuing the facts of a child's life reveals much about their functioning and pulls patients into the gears of therapy.

Knowing what stresses and stressors are ongoing also puts the referral complaint into a broader picture. That parents are discussing divorce at home may explain Cindy's sliding grades more than the bad influence of her new boyfriend, as cited by her mother. Marital tensions, births and deaths, illnesses, financial shifts, moves, and changes at school are a sampling of the circumstances that can precipitate new problems and symptoms or motivate the referral for problems and symptoms that have existed for a while.

If the child is suffering, we spend time trying to find out the precise nature of the angst. When and how much does it hurt? What makes it worse, and what seems to soothe it? When did it begin? Does it ever get unbearable? Do the anxiety and depression seem directly related to a recent incident or dilemma, or are they more entrenched? Does the pain seem to have neurotic meaning, a young girl's body expressing her reluctance to separate? Does it appear to be a sign of more serious illness? Or is this a child, we ask ourselves, who must dramatically hurt to gain the sympathy and nurturing of a self-absorbed mother?

What about the child's general health? This question is especially important for children who come with bodily aches for which doctors can't find a cause. "What happens when you think you're dying?" I've asked a young girl with stomachaches, before turning to ask her mother,

"What happens when you think your daughter's dying? Who are her doctors? How have they managed the child? What has worked and what hasn't? How does Julie feel about doctors anyway?" I ask. Although I suspect with some certainty that the child's psyche has everything to do with her distress, I explore this area with the same care and thought that guides my queries into the medical life of children coping with chronic and well-documented illness.

I eventually obtain a developmental history, although not in the first session or two. When were milestones achieved? Which ones came precociously, and which came late? Have there been separations or other potentially stressing circumstances? How parents negotiate these questions can reveal more than the answers themselves.

We inquire about previous treatment. If other clinicians have been involved, we want to know when and for how long and for what reason they were consulted. "Did it help?" I ask the child. "Did it help?" I ask the parents, following up both with a why or why not. "Did you consider returning to Dr. Black?" I'll ask, perplexed that parents came to me, given their and their child's stated esteem for her. Although parents escaping from other therapists may flatter us, we can't help but wonder what makes them (and us) think that we'll succeed where, perhaps, other competent clinicians have not.

Cultural and ethnic background are also of great relevance. The meanings of our questions, the meanings of behaviors and symptoms, the meanings of relationships, and the meanings of seeking help and therapy vary among cultures. Some patients are guarded with therapists of a different color or faith. However, assuming that my being green and a worshipper of the star Crypto gives me complete and reliable understanding of every Martian is a mistake. To share a culture or heritage does not guarantee our knowing the private and individual family culture in which a child lives.

However difficult, by the end of the second if not the first hour, I ask virtually all parents whether, to their knowledge, anyone in their child's life abuses alcohol, drugs, or the child—physically or sexually. If asked without fanfare and apprehension, I've found most parents willing to reply, even when the answers are not happy ones. For the few who are unwilling, their running or less frantic refusal can be the beginning of an answer to what we've asked.

Most of what we learn is told to us spontaneously or in response to what we say and ask. But we can also glean much information by subtler means, such as observing what we see. From the minute our door swings open, our search begins. Does the child appear well cared for, well fed, rosy-cheeked, and dressed for the weather? Our worrimeters can't help but go off when we meet a first-grade boy who has black-and-blue bags under his eyes or who wears shorts and a T-shirt on this nippy late autumn morning. Although I may discover soon enough that he is a wayward student, finding a new patient doing his algebra in the waiting room encourages me. Finding that a child has tipped over the magazine table and is now taking apart the thermostat does not.

We watch the children walk and move about the office. Do they trip and bump their way across the room, or do they enter gracefully? Do they sit comfortably or fidget? I note to myself the blinking tic of one boy and the natural calm of a second. How do they hold and use a crayon? Some children cover the table with an intricate knockdown in the time it takes another to successfully stand six dominoes. "How does this work?" a slow 10-year-old may ask out of frustration, about to snap a simple twist-to-use pen, whereas the next patient, a first grader, takes it upon himself to correctly adjust the time on a complicated office clock. And, of course, who can miss easy grins, forced smiles, flushed humiliation, and sometimes the saddest faces that lie flat, doing nothing at all. These data, too numerous to imagine or mention, bombard us and allow us to unobtrusively assess varied aspects of the child, such as how coordinated, tense, confident, assertive, able to withstand frustration, energetic, self-protective, and happy he is.

Such observable data can take strange forms. Seeing an adolescent boy pull a handful of dried peas (*where's the slingshot?*), carelessly crumpled paper (*the print looks like something to do with school?*), too much money (*where did he get it, or what's he need it for?*), and a butane lighter (*to smoke, to light fires?*) out of his pocket leads me to question his risk for delinquency, his judgment, and his need to show it off to me. (In this case, he wanted help with his impulsivity.)

And think of the four-year-old who carefully blew her stuffed-up nose, managing the entire hour with one tissue. "Excuse me," she said, covering a dainty sneeze with her hand. Compare her with the first grader who, waving off my offer for even one sheet, wiped his snot over his overalls and my chair when he wasn't coughing fountains of spit over my desk and glasses. We can't draw conclusions from such sparse data, nor can we assume that the more hygienic girl was better adjusted and parented (though she was). But we surely can start to know who these children are.

We generally don't need to ask a lot of odd and distracting questions. Listening to what children say, whatever they say, can show us whether they are oriented in time and space and whether they can discern outer from inner reality. The sound, style, pace, structure, and vocabulary of their speech, if heeded, can alert us to their cognitive functioning and learning experiences, especially involving language. Clarity and coherence of thought is obvious in an hour's worth of interview, as is the child's ability to listen and understand us. Is the child especially concrete, eccentrically vague and abstract, or does she fluidly go between the two appropriately for a child that age? We can do much of a neurological assessment with little effort and ruckus.

We learn, too, from watching the child interact with his family. Although a reasonable level of communication, respect, and affection doesn't ensure that all is well at home, I prefer that to a family that marches in coldly, sharing neither a glance nor a word among themselves. In my experience, friendly teasing, particularly genuine smiles and self-disparagement, often goes along with better put together families; biting sarcasm, hostile put-downs, and blaming of others frequently does not.

Who sits where and with whom? Why do my young patient—referred around a learning disability—and her toddler sister cling to their mother's arms while their father sits passively alone across the room? Do they like her more? Is he somehow toxic or uninvolved? Frightened by the interview, do they seek their mother for security? Or maybe she's a narcissistic woman who demands her daughters' attention and audience, ignoring their wish to be near their dad? By taking note now and as time and events pass, we learn the motives behind what we see. In this case, the dynamic proved rather simply, pleasantly, and humbly surprising. The children had missed their mother. She'd just returned from a three-day trip to care for an elderly aunt. Their father, having spent every hour of the past long weekend with them, was pooped.

Do the parents listen to the young boy? Do they respect his opinion? Do they treat him like a child his age, one much older, a baby, or, painfully, like an object? If both parents are present, how do they treat one another? Is the child preferred greatly by one parent and disliked by the other? Does the child seem to be more the wife to her father than does her mother?

How the boy treats his family is no less informative. Does he listen and show respect, or does he cruelly bully his caring, if ineffective mother? One mildly jealous boy tripped his sister on the way into the office. Another, much more dangerously jealous, devoted his hour to slavishly waiting on his little brother, trying, he later confessed, to deceive me with his over-done show of concern. Every interaction, big or small, carries clues about the child and the social fabric in which she lives and was formed.

Perhaps our most useful source of data is the child's way of being with us. Is eye contact comfortable or hollow, or does the child avoid our gaze as if our own eyes are the halogen headlights of an oncoming truck? Does the child speak with and otherwise treat us like a human being, seeming to have empathy for us and to notice the empathy we have for him? Or might the therapist just as well be a computer or robot that the child manipulates with a keyboard or remote control? Keeping the child's age and language development in mind, is there give-and-take in our conversation?

Is he trusting and friendly, or does he, as did one eighth grader, ward me off with a barrage of insults (which, being mostly about my stupidity and queerness, revealed his two biggest fears about himself)? Children, while talking, have occasionally dedicated their hour to neatening my office, handling the stress of the meeting with helpful and conciliatory behavior. Just as commonly, children test me with their uncooperative demeanor, deliberately messing my desk or casually dropping a candy wrapper on the floor with an eye toward my reaction.

What are the child's emotions? Are they assorted and understandable? Are they varied but muted, like a subdued foliage season, or do they come and go with the speed and power of lightning? Does depression or mania prevail? Are his feelings in keeping and proportion with what he is saying? If not, do they betray feelings near the surface, as did one boy's hostility while telling of his pleasure at receiving a much desired birthday gift? Or is the discrepancy between affect and content more worrisome? I've met too many like the sociopathic teenager who couldn't contain his categorical pleasure while describing the skinning of a squirrel he'd killed with a stone. We may meet more seriously ill children whose affect and facial expression are somehow strange or seem wholly stuck or lacking.

Although the data the child offers are virtually unlimited, I am most interested in the child's honesty with me. When a child admits to remorse, regret, self-hatred, or a wish to change—*and means it*—I am singularly encouraged that therapy will help. A rigid externalizing of responsibility, blaming everyone but herself, worries me.

Assuming we have a good sense of ourselves, how we feel with patients can be a treasure chest of data. A boy talked with glee about the space ride at the county fair, yet I felt an overwhelming sadness. (His mother later told me that he saw his divorced father there with another woman.) And what accounted for my feeling increasingly indifferent to a charming 15-year-old girl's horrid tale of abuse? (I soon found that her intentionally groomed extroversion barely hid a profound vulnerability to dissociate.)

It is my own unexpected or seemingly out-of-line reactions that alert me to something special about what's going on with the child. Needless to say, when using ourselves and our feelings in this way, we must beware of confusing our own unresolved issues and blind spots with those of our patients. The greater experience and self-knowledge we gain by doing therapy, receiving supervision, being in therapy, and continually reflecting on our work generally enhances the reliability of our intuiting.[1]

FORMULATING AND DIAGNOSING

From that virtually limitless sea of clues, we begin to put together a puzzle that is the child. But it isn't the rectangular puzzles we are used to building with our own children. This puzzle has no frame, no flat pieces to set us straight on our path, and it can be almost any shape. Being good at this kind of puzzle requires that we be flexible in our thinking. We need sufficient energy and motivation to try each clue, seeing where it best fits, often setting it aside, alongside thousands of other clues, to be sorted and tried again and again, eventually finding its right place or falling into uselessness.

It is in this intellectually demanding enterprise that theory and facts collide. If we go forth into the consulting room as pure empiricists, persuaded only by what we see, we will be exquisitely open to every possibility. Yet without any theory or hypotheses about how children work, we may find ourselves immobilized by the volume of information or doing therapy by the seat of our pants, reacting more than deliberating.

Being too convinced of our theories, can also retard our work. Believing that we know what has to be can deceive us, leading us to see only the data that support our theories. Holding on to our theories too rigidly, we are prone to force data into our thinking rather than using data to inform and guide what we think. It was that kind of intellectual posture that, at its worst, caused well-meaning clinicians to tragically and destructively see "innocent" mothers as agents of their children's autism by having withheld love and nurturing. Clinicians tend to run to their theories when most stressed, confused, or lost—precisely the times when more openness and vision are called for. And so as responsible clinicians, we seek a balance, one that is fluid, that can accommodate and assimilate, and that can grow as we learn and experience more of therapy and more of life.

Even with the most well-equilibrated perspective, our task is daunting. Finding a *DSM-IV* (American Psychiatric Association, 2000) diagnosis is easy enough. But what does that tell and do for us? That freckled red-headed boy who sidled up beside me—affectionately showing me his pet frog, tearful about the polluting of the ponds, missing his divorced father, dreading that I'll bring up his bed-wetting, tortured by his nightmares, struggling with his reading, frustrated by a congenital hip dysfunction, jealous about his younger sister, fearful of his anger, more fearful of being rejected, and worried that his mother has been very tired lately—absolutely and positively, just no way can be neatly stuffed into a jar labeled "307.6 Enuresis," "315.00 Reading Disorder," "300.2 Overanxious Disorder of Childhood," or even the more generous and forgiving "309.0 Adjustment Disorder."[2]

When formulating who a child is, we strive to put the presenting problems into a deservingly complex context that includes all the information we have collected in the first meetings. Only when we begin to know who the child is can we begin to understand the meaning, reasons, and causes of his symptoms and behaviors—and the likely best method to help. Using our good clinical sense, we review our inventory to formally answer more questions concerning the child's intellect, health, reality testing, ego functioning, object relatedness, development of self, conscience, school adjustment, peer relations, family dynamics, and environmental circumstances, both stressing and supporting. Although these psychological terms may intimidate us, as may their demand that we organize our data clinically, by this time we have more than enough information to do what we must.

GIVING PARENTS AND THEIR CHILD FEEDBACK

When, after a number of sessions, we feel that we have seen both child and parents enough to have a good, if beginning, sense of things, we meet with the parents and their child—sometimes together, sometimes apart—to tell them what we think. We include the young girl for the obvious reason that she is the one coming, the one we are talking about. She came to our meetings and fulfilled her part of the bargain. She's entitled to hear our serious and well-considered assessment of what she's experiencing.

Children and parents are vulnerable when awaiting the expert's judgment. We generally begin by asking what they most fear hearing. "That she's crazy." "That he's going to be a serial killer." "That he's never going to be happy." Parents' questions about their children often reveal deep dreads and guilt.

This reminds us of the need to choose our words carefully. We have to tell things as they are. But we have great latitude in how we share what we've learned and, in sadder times, how we break the news. Comparing Johnny's brain to a "broken and poorly wired computer" is apt to arouse despair, as would coldly telling them that their child is abnormal.

There *are* better ways. We can use words that people know and understand. Explaining in detail how Cliff wishes to be loved exclusively and that his disruptive antics are intended more to gain affection than to inflict hurt will do more than glibly referring to his oedipal conflicts. Saying, "When Elaine faces a difficult task, she avoids humiliation by daydreaming of being a supermodel" does what "Elaine has attention deficit disorder" cannot. Doesn't describing how a child doesn't do something so well in certain situations beat a vague reference to his dysfunction?

We respect the value of clarity, which nearly every book on the craft of writing extols. When an author writes obscurely, worships big words, overuses the passive voice, and gets lost in endless sentences that say little, there's a good chance that he's not sure what he wants to say. Whether out of insecurity or fear, some clinicians state their findings so tentatively and with so much qualifying that it's hard to know what they've said.

We tell parents and their child almost anything we feel is of value, and we try particularly to explain the possible meanings of the referring complaint and the strengths and weaknesses that the child and family bring to that issue. When we must share our sense that something is seriously amiss, we don't rush to get it over, blurting out "mental illness." We go slowly, our care itself warning parents that something is coming and giving them time to begin processing what we'll be telling them. We do not speak first of *psychosis* but instead describe the difficulty their child has distinguishing outer reality from what he imagines, elaborating how this varies under different stresses as well as ways in which it has been adaptive and protective. Our efforts are not to avoid something bad; they are meant to avoid shocking a parent with one awful word so they become unable to hear and understand anything further. After a lengthy discussion of what a lack-of-reality testing means for their child, for example, it is not unusual for a parent to then ask if that is what *psychotic* means, a question we then answer directly in the affirmative.

When parents take the blame unfairly for their child's problems—such as autism or a learning disability—we try to offset their self-criticism. But in cases where parenting and home life have been detrimental, we neither lobby for their self-forgiveness nor rush to relieve their guilt. Nor do we make light of their having delayed treatment for years.[3]

After sharing our sense of what's going on, we address what therapy can do. Here again our work is challenging. Father may want a better behaved Tony. Mother may want a happier Tony. School may want a harder-working Tony. Tony wants a more confident Tony and one whom his parents will like more. Everyone's vision of goals is relevant here, and usually they are compatible.

Short-term goals versus long term. Big goals versus little. Inner goals versus outer. Do we want symptom relief, changed behavior, more insight, better self-control, increased resilience, more connectedness, or just a more cooperative daughter?

When offering treatment, we do not promise the world—sometimes because we don't think it will be forthcoming, more often because only time and therapy will tell. But neither do we prematurely predict what may never happen. I have worked with too many children whose parents were told—wrongly, time proved—that their child would never ride a bicycle or drive a car (he is a skilled cyclist and driver), never succeed in even the lowliest classroom (as she came out of her cocoon she showed herself to be gifted and is now a college student), never throw a ball (became a varsity athlete), never relate to friends like other children (became a class officer), and never work at anything (now an earnest and self-motivated lobbyist for the environment). Gloomy predictions seldom add anything, especially at an early age.

Once we offer treatment, we do not push parents or children to make a decision on the spot. We watch for signs of ambivalence or confusion and meet them head-on. We know that sweeping such tensions under the rug will not get rid of them and may lead to bigger resistances later on. "Of course you are unsure about this whole idea," I easily said to one skeptical father. "Bringing your child to a therapist is a strange business." Accepted in his uncertainty, this father was then able to reveal his own bad experience with a therapist years ago as well as his current fear that I might do badly by his son.

When parents agree to bring their child to us for therapy, they have entrusted us with their most cherished possession. At the very least, all of our assessing and interacting with the child and her parents up to this point should attest to our recognizing the privilege and responsibility of that decision.[4]

NOTES

1. As Frederick Allen said more than 40 years ago in his chapter "The Beginning Phase of Therapy" (in Haworth, 1964), the "degree to which the immediate behavior of the child is utilized in this beginning phase is influenced by the particular therapeutic approach" (p. 103). Psychodynamic therapists want to see it all—words, nonverbal behaviors, resistances, and so on—as a welcome part and parcel of the work. Likewise, as the client-centered Allen states, "Beginning where the child actually is and dealing directly and immediately with his feelings, rather than with his problem behavior and its causes, give an immediate impetus and meaning to the therapeutic process" (p. 104). He goes on to poignantly and, in my view, accurately emphasize, "Therapy is a precipitated growth experience, not apart from but akin to life."

What I call "getting to know" the child, of course, technically equals assessment, an evaluation that starts from the first hello. Psychodynamic practitioners seek an enormous amount of data that tell us about current functioning, symptoms, ego strength, intellectual skills, spontaneity and range of mood, health, relationships, social engagement, socioeconomic status, and so on. Because the (potential) therapeutic process also begins at hello, we tend not to want to burden or obstruct the child with too much structure or a litany of boxed questions. And so we train ourselves to be subversive and unobtrusive gatherers of information who can take it all in without 101 pointed questions.

Cognitive-behavioral clinicians and other short-term practitioners generally waste neither time nor attention following a child's associations, detours, or resistances. Interpersonal nuances, such as what the interacting with the child feels like, might be considered more static than inroad. These clinicians often follow a strict agenda and regimen that includes a clear-cut and economical time line. As a result, by the end of the first hour, these clinicians—by some combination of direct child and/or parent interview and behavioral checklists—may have collected enough data to initiate their therapeutic programs.

2. A fair discussion of the merits and flaws of *DSM-IV(TR)* is far beyond the scope and space of this book. Although such a system has its place—that is, can be justified for reasons of insurance, research, communication, and epidemiology—it doesn't always do great justice to individuals and their treatments. As I wrote elsewhere (Bromfield, 1996), "ADHD exists as a disorder," for example, "primarily because a committee voted it so" (p. 26), a human enterprise lent some worry and credence by a recent finding that a majority of committee members have some connection to the pharmaceutical companies that profit from these disorders—including direct financial ties (56 percent), research support (42 percent), and consulting fees (22 percent) (Cosgrove & Krimsky, 2006). Although this doesn't invalidate their decision making, make diagnosis a useless or obsolete effort, or negate the substantial value of psychotropic medication, it does caution us to proceed with eyes wide open. We know that our field is prone to fads, an exaggerated exuberance that can unfortunately trounce the prudent guidelines set forth for a disorder's identification and treatment. The concepts of a self-fulfilling prophecy and a viciously downward spiral bear relevance here. Diagnoses can take on lives of their own, distracting and detouring clinicians, teachers, and parents from other ways of thinking and intervening that, in the long run, might help reverse or remediate a condition thought to be irrevocable.

As to the usefulness of *DSM-IV(TR)* diagnosis versus formulation, consider Lenore Terr's (2006) stimulating inquiry. She wrote clinicians asking for detailed vignettes of turnaround moments in children's and teenagers' therapies. A majority of them suggested that there exist critical "moments" or juncture in a therapy when treating by formulation outweighs treating by diagnosis. This, of course, does not represent a scientific study of the issue as much as it suggests the need for more and stronger research. Moreover, we can easily imagine examples where treating diagnosis and formulation are not at odds.

3. Here, too, the clinician's theoretical orientation determines much of how feedback will be given. Although most all clinicians strive to be tactful and compassionate, our frames of reference will determine the ways we offer our observations. A psychodynamic or child-centered child therapist may wish to describe a whole child in a form that clearly and accurately portrays

the child in all her glorious complexity. While more behavioral clinicians may approach the child with equal kindness and warmth, they may therapeutically cut to the chase, describing the child and her issues with a succinctness and singularity to match the treatment.

4. The concept of offering treatment may seem rather unrealistic to clinicians who work in clinics, schools, and so on where they are assigned patients to treat, period. Even in that more restricted scenario, however, considering and contemplating these dynamics can only increase the likelihood that child and parents will not drop out of therapy.

3

The Not-So-Magic of Therapy: How Therapy Works

Psychotherapy can appear to be a rather strange and mysterious business. Some see us as doing our good or bad by some form of psychic voodoo, exerting a magical influence on another's mind. Many, even some clinicians, judge that, for all of our fancy theory and prices, we help mostly by being a good friend to someone who's hurting or confused. What, in fact, does therapy do, and how does it do it?

MAKING A SAFE PLACE

The issue of safety is one that underlies so many aspects of what happens in treatment. Why would anyone, no less a child, want to spend time with or maybe even open up or grow close to someone who posed a danger?

> In his first four sessions 14-year-old Kevin wore an oversized turtle-neck stretched over his lower face. Through this cotton veil, his

muffled voice spoke about his "stupid, ugly teachers," the "stupid, ugly girls" in his class, and his "stupid, ugly parents." He even put down the "stupid, ugly" dog he saw outside my office (a neighbor's bright and handsome, if jumpy, golden retriever), seeming to have no awareness of just how frequently he used those precise and demeaning words. Knowing from his mother that Kevin believed his chin was somehow misshapen, his self-consciousness making daily life an unbearable ordeal, I did not push his face into what he said or what he wore, but instead patiently waited.

In his fifth hour Kevin asked me if I knew why he hid his face. Neither surprised nor bothered by my affirming nod, he expressed gratitude that I'd let him be the one to bring up the subject. "You know," he added, pulling his turtleneck down for the first time, "I just tripped over the dog, and she's really not ugly at all."

My respect for his guardedness made Kevin feel safe enough to bring up the real reason he was here, a chin that, while hardly monstrous, had become a repository for his seeing himself as the stupid and ugly one. My waiting allowed Kevin, in his own time, to take ownership of his reason for coming and to voluntarily join forces with me and the therapy. Without such therapeutic allying—a process that grows and grows throughout a sound course of therapy—we therapists are essentially controlling masters who push and pull our stubborn donkeys along the trail.

To do therapy requires that a child look at herself. Our looking at her, though helpful, is not enough. But to look at herself, she must expose her most precious goods—what she thinks, feels, does, says, plays, and draws—putting her at risk of the therapist's ridicule, rejection, or otherwise negative reaction. Although we might stand on our desks and loudly proclaim that we would never ever do such things, it is only our unwavering acceptance—in good and bad and over time—that will convince her she is in trustworthy company.

For the traumatized child, the safety of therapy provides an immediate shelter, a place where she can't be hurt or abused for the moment and, perhaps, ever again. She needs first to be rescued from harm's way. Only when safe from abuse and neglect can she—and we—afford to look at the damage and begin restoring what we can. Only when she knows she is no longer in danger can she start to make sense of her experience. Her soiled trust, like that of any abused child, must be earned back. As long as we live in a house made of straw or mud, we should be wary of the wolf. Unfortunately for children whose love and trust have been betrayed or who have suffered more random violence or tragedy, even walls of brick and steel do not make for feelings of security. The haven of therapy serves increasingly as a fortress in which the child can work on better understanding and growing past her trauma.

The safety of therapy can let a mildly hampered child catch his breath. The nonjudgmental atmosphere of therapy gradually invites children to let down not just their hair but their swords and shields, too. "Geez, what a relief," said one big bully some weeks after having shared that he's petrified of insects. He'd found a place where he could start to be himself.

Throughout treatment, especially for those who for too long have held on to stress or pain, the safety of therapy allows for catharsis and abreaction, the letting go of feelings. Some children will hold on to their tears for weeks while remembering Muffin or their grandfather, their faces crunched, their eyes swollen red, their brows quivering, feeling that boys shouldn't cry or that, once begun, they'll never be able to stop. But when they cry, they usually feel better. Although sobbing and wailing in themselves do not make for a treatment and generally do not lead to growth, they can relieve a great deal of pressure and sometimes bring unexpected insights.

> Laura's parents had brought the 13-year-old because she was sleeping poorly, eating little, and not seeming her cheery self. A few weeks into therapy it was already clear that Laura—good student, daughter, and friend—was the salt of the earth. Why, she would even take her retarded younger sister with her to the mall. "If kids don't have room in their hearts for her, then I don't have room in mine for them," Laura told me.
>
> Not knowing where this might lead, I didn't praise the goodness that was so evident. This proved to be sound when Laura, months later—talking about receiving a helping award from the Special Olympics—suddenly began crying. "What is it, Laura?" I asked.
>
> "I'm a rotten person," she wailed. "I'm not at all the good girl people think I am. It's me that should have been born retarded. It's me that should be dead."

What Laura meant, we came to see, went further than her survivor guilt, her having intellectual gifts that her sister did not. The thought that she "deserved to die," that she be sentenced to death, came from an even darker place. "Sometimes I wish she were dead," Laura finally gasped between sobs. "I don't want to spend my whole life taking care of her," she explained. "I don't want to spend my whole life feeling bad 'cause I'm not retarded, too." As long as Laura had held back her tears, she was able to hold back the pained sentiment behind them.[1]

The refuge of therapy, including the therapist's steady presence, can allow a child to grieve a recent loss. That loss need not be a death but can be the unavailability of or profound disappointment in a person or the loss of a child's ideals of what she or life should be. Often—and with more difficulty—that same refuge can permit a delayed or stunted bereaving to reawaken, surface, and pass. Not uncommonly, children who save their mourning are children who temperamentally tend to hold in their feelings or who come from homes where sadness cannot be tolerated.

The dependable quiet and calm of therapy is particularly critical to the work for children who are easily overstimulated. An overly cluttered office and, even worse, an overly cluttered therapist run the risk of maintaining the distractible child in overdrive, obstructing his use of treatment. For the thin-skinned child, the emotional insulation of therapy—meaning mostly that the therapist expects nothing much from the patient and keeps his own feelings to himself—is itself reparative. Like turtles midst a flock of seagulls, such children, sensing danger everywhere, remain in their shells, lest they be forced into contact with people and their feelings. Only by allowing them to keep their shells on for protection and security do they eventually stick their necks and heads out.

Providing this insulating function can be tough work for the therapist. Work with high-functioning autistic or Asperger children shows how difficult it is to give a child all the aloneness he needs. To truly feel what this child feels about us means feeling unneeded, unwanted, noxious, dangerous, and as having needs and feelings that the child deeply does not want to be around. Yet if we force ourselves on the child, we can lose her for a long time, if not forever.[2]

The safety of the office offers traumatized children repeated opportunity to begin mastering their tragic and sometimes dehumanizing experiences. But again, supplying that stable setting isn't easy.

Russell, a sixth-grade boy whose utter lack of self-confidence clashed with his good brains, looks, and musical talents, was oblivious to me.

He intently pushed the end of one paper clip into the other, over and over, in and out, until, remembering I was there, with embarrassment he threw the clips into the wastebasket. Some weeks later he brought his own jumbo clip to sadistically jam it through the middle of a normal-sized paper clip. Russell elaborated this activity—jabbing pencils, soda bottles, and then his fingers into big globs of clay, until, one day, shocked by his having stuck a pencil into my couch, he confessed having been molested by a male babysitter as a young child.

I knew he'd been abused before we'd ever met; his parents had told me. He and I had even discussed it during the first meetings. But he'd forgotten—he had to. I knew enough to know that Russell's belabored preoccupation with paper clips and stabbing carried significance and needed to be given room for its expression. Fortunately, I was secure enough to tolerate the feelings that expression (and all that it implied) evoked. Had I been repulsed, frightened, or in some other way uncomfortable with what I'd learned, I likely could not have preserved the therapeutic space so well, likely distracting both of us with observations about his aggression or unrelated issues or asking questions about, perhaps, his schoolwork.

The safe space we create also allows for the playing out of developmental tasks in the service of their mastery.

"Well, I'm going now. I'm leaving home," five-year-old Ginger said sweetly for the moose puppet.

"Goodbye," I said, watching Ginger's arm hide the moose behind her back. But he wasn't gone for long.

"Surprise!" Ginger exclaimed, the moose suddenly back in my face.

"How nice to see you again!"

"Gee, it's great to be back," Ginger's moose replied. "But I think I have to leave again. Bye." And so it went, on each trip moose going farther away and for a longer time.

Five-year-old Ginger wanted to go to kindergarten but she didn't like leaving her home. Her mom, having lost her own mother when in early elementary school, had comparable doubts about Ginger's going off. But Ginger's play suggested that her wish to go was greater than her fear. A rather healthy child from a good home who sensed the safety of my office and me, Ginger spontaneously went to work in her first session.

In a handful of hours, Ginger's reenacting of a moose–child's leave-taking and rapprochement cleared the way for an open discussion of her worry that being a big girl at school might cost her some dependency and nurturing. She soon was off and running.

In a similar fashion, children who feel small, helpless, and otherwise powerless in the face of big and little insults use the permissive and secure aspect of therapy to revise history. In her play, a real-life victim can cast herself as a hero. A good girl, who outside therapy lacked any appreciation for her less-than-holy thoughts, plays an evil witch. Perpetually beat up and made fun of by his older brother, a boy comes in weekly to be the tyrant. More than a few children play school, notoriously assuming the role of bossy teacher. By being the one in control, children come to better understand and cope with the many life situations in which they must bend to authority and rules.

The ways by which the sanctuary we create enables and furthers a course of therapy are as numerous as they are indispensable. No one has taught us these core principles better than the client-centered school of child therapy. For example, read the instructive, lively, and rich work of Virginia Axline (1947, 1964), Haim Ginott (1959, 1961, 1968), and Clark Moustakas (1959). However, contrary to their view, I do not think that a nonthreatening, nonjudging, and nondirecting atmosphere, while imperative, is enough for most children's therapies. Children will indeed unfold and blossom when given the psychic equivalents of sunlight, water, and rich soil, but only to a point. Most of us, children included, have blind spots, conflicts, trauma, and other vulnerabilities that we hide and protect even in what appear to be the most open and welcoming of settings. Even in the arms of the kindest of therapists, children need to be confronted, informed, or otherwise acted on to find relief and move ahead.[3]

HOLDING

Perhaps the most basic, powerful, and yet difficult function we serve is to hold our patients.

> "I'm going to eat my shit out of myself and then stuff it in my mother's breasts and shoot her and me on an alien ship to Pluto and then come back and then and then I'm and then I'm going to stuff my head in

a dog's ass and walk to school, barking at everybody, and peeing on
their shoes, and when my spaceship gets back from Pluto me and my
mom will have a baby that drinks acid and likes to eat toxic waste and
it'll grow real big and it'll do sex with everybody and . . ."

Drew's soliloquy moved nonstop and at the speed of light. Each metaphor grew more divergent and disturbing than the last. If I had bailed
out on him, simply admitting that what he spoke of and his deteriorating
state was too much for me, no one would have faulted me. Previous clinicians had judged him to be too ill to be helped by outpatient therapy.

They were wrong. With just weekly meetings, he'd managed in regular schools for the previous two years and had become dramatically less
hostile, aggressive, and susceptible to stress. In my view, this more recent
regression was a positive sign that he was bringing his more crazed self
into the treatment, something he'd previously shown more outside of
the therapy office.

". . . And then and then the baby is going to grow a big dick and shove
it everywhere and bite his crib and eat his crib and his Popeye mobile
and then he's going to fly into the sky and fly back to earth . . ."

Drew neither halted his story nor behaviorally broke down. I could see
that he was not truly out of control but was sharing something important, however intense and undifferentiated.

"And then he's going to poop and poop and poop more poop than
everyone's ever seen, all over his school. No one's going to be able to
find the school it'll be so lost in that mountain of crap."

By the end of the session, Drew quieted. And so had his story. I was
not afraid of his words or the primitive impulses and thinking behind
them. I did little but listen. I didn't interrupt, nor did I distract him.
I didn't stop to question him about sexual abuse, suicidal ideation, or his
relationship with his mother. I knew he functioned at home and school.
I didn't take his psychotic-sounding ranting as a sign that he needed
inpatient treatment (whatever that is these days).

"School. A school covered in poop," I said aloud, aware that the final
and more coherent words probably carried the message, if there was
one. "Is something going on in school?"

There was, Drew told me. Lots. A failed spelling exam. Being embarrassed by a teacher's flippant remark. Tripping to the floor in gym. But more than everything Drew was panicked over a school project for which he was giving a small talk the next day—a talk that, to his and my surprise, went uneventfully well.

By emotionally containing Drew—"You don't get freaked out by my crazy stuff like everyone else does"—I allowed him to feel and express without having to bear the burden of hurting, terrifying, or repelling me and without the fear of being punished or hospitalized for exposing himself. My steady presence in the wake of his explosion somewhat detoxified the awful things that tormented his insides. By sharing the horrendous ways in which he feared losing self-control, ways that held sane and understandable meaning, he actually came to have more control over himself.

Although we don't cradle our patients physically, we hold our patients like mothers do their babies. When our patients are colicky or overstimulated with anger or irritation, we stay right with them, calming them with *our* calm, using ourselves, like sponges, to absorb and regulate some of the affect that torments them. That the most petite of woman therapists can comfort and contain the brawniest of male patients demonstrates the psychological power of our holding. Although a wild and enormous teenager may know that I could never single-handedly restrain him—bigger adults in his life have tried—he somehow feels safe with me, meaning safe from himself, his thoughts, and what he might do.[4]

We can hold our patients in relation to almost any feeling or worry, lending them ego that they, at least for the moment, are missing. For example, ninth-grader Bobby came to a session angry enough to kill another child who'd ridiculed him in front of a prospective girlfriend. By sharing his rage with me, he came to his own senses, saw more clearly why he was so incensed, and came up with a solution that needn't hurt himself or his rival. Our holding can help restore and integrate children who lack personal definition or are prone to fragment under stress.

The therapist's holding, although concentrated at certain points (such as during a panic or in a phase where suicidal thinking is prominent), occupies most every moment of every sound therapy. It helps our patients to tolerate and face the therapeutic work and discomfort without having to flee, disintegrate, or attack. While especially important for child patients whose parents are unwilling or unable to hold them (because of

their own deficits or as a result of a mismatch with their child's temperament), it matters even to the child from a high-functioning and nur-
turant home. In the best of treatments, this holding—an inner sense that
we and therapy are with them—endures beyond the office walls, helping
our patients to function, cope, stay out of trouble, and suffer less for the
six days and 23 or so hours when they are without us.

INTERVENING

Just as holding psychologically replicates an aspect of the mother–child
relationship, other therapeutic functions also both borrow from and seek
to promote natural and good human development. Mothers mirror what
their young children think and feel, and we try to do the same with our
patients. "You really are sad today" or "You don't want me telling your
parents" confirms our patients' experiences, helping to solidify their own
convictions. Our getting it right and making it clear—meaning genuinely, not by rote or empty parroting—is most valuable to the child who
has been raised to rely not on her own thoughts and feelings but rather
on those of a narcissistically fragile parent. But this applies to all children
in therapy, for they all have aspects of themselves that are less authentic
than others, areas in which they are less trusting of their own perceptions
and sentiments.

Parents tend to admire and take pleasure in their children's growth,
shaky first steps, and adorable first words. As therapists we too encourage
our patients by noting their courage in doing therapy and taking pride in
their efforts. "How brave of you, Molly," I said to a girl who, rather than
start a fight with her classmates, shared the underlying frustration with
her teacher. Therapy often intercedes in areas where decent parents have
been unable to celebrate their child's developing, for example, a loving
mother who, herself fearful of separation, rejects her child whenever he
takes a healthy giant step toward independence or a compulsively clean
father who rejects his dear son's adventurousness because of the dirt and
bugs that come along. The satisfaction that we as therapists derive from
our patients' progress and efforts helps to revive their developmental
momentum in those blocked areas.

Empathy, a hallmark of the good child–parent relationship, is also crucial to effective psychotherapy. More than walking in another's shoes or
taking his perspective, empathy means understanding and conveying that

you understand another's feelings or situation. Sometimes we demon-strate our empathy in our heartfelt reflecting, "It's just so discouraging." Sometimes we empathize by doing things, such as handing a box of tis-sues to a child whose eyes are welling, our gesture saying, "It's okay, you can cry." At other times, realizing that our words aren't wanted or won't be helpful, we empathize by means of our silent presence or by nodding good-bye instead of exuberantly wishing a good week. Any manner of intervening that is intimately sensitive to where the child is emotionally and to what she needs is empathic.

The feeling of empathy, of being understood, is one we all enjoy and want and one that can itself heal, especially for the child who doesn't get enough of it. Letting a misbehaving and defensive child know that *his* plight is understood ("You feel picked on by everybody") can help him to let his other-blaming guard down and look at what he might have done.

Our steady empathy throughout therapy serves not only to bathe the child in understanding but also to set the stage for the many and inevitable moments when we misunderstand the child. These lapses, so-called *empathic failures,* offer some of the most therapeutically power-ful opportunities in a course of treatment.

> "I said something wrong, didn't I?" I spoke just loud enough to be heard. But no response came from under the chair where Brian had curled himself up. His trombone lay on the floor where he'd dropped it and himself one instant after I'd praised his playing. He'd come to therapy directly from school band rehearsal. A perfectionistic and brit-tley shy child, even his agreeing to do band was a major victory. Even more striking was his suggesting that he play a concert for me.
>
> The session passed with Brian in his "cave." In the final minutes he spoke. "I played awful and you know it. Why'd you say I played nicely? That's like making fun of me."

However well intentioned, my words that he'd played nicely did any-thing but make Brian feel good. If we'd stopped there, Brian would have left feeling worse and smaller than when he came, cursing the moment he'd decided to bring his instrument along. But we didn't.

With my urging, Brian reflected on his performance. He acknowl-edged comparing his playing to that of his accomplished teacher rather than a standard fitting a novice trombonist. Brian assumed that I was as disappointed in his playing as he was. He saw how his injured pride and image of himself had led to his withdrawing, which brought a long inch of growth to his becoming less self-criticizing and less likely to quit activities that he enjoyed. Over the course of Brian's therapy, its many empathic failures and their repair brought him increased and lasting resiliency against the slings and arrows that pervaded his daily life.[5]

It is our empathy that enables us to gauge where children are in terms of tension and affect so that we intervene at the proper time and to the right degree. We seek to push them to deal with as much as they adaptively can. To overwhelm children's resources is counterproductive and can set them back; to underwhelm them supports the status quo, inviting regression and complacency. By titrating how much we emotionally confront children—ever striving to provide the optimal amount of intervention—we psychically stretch them. This slow and steady work exercises children's capacities to tolerate and manage their emotions, making them less irritable and less impulsive.[6]

Ultimately, much of therapy is motivated by a hope for change. But people must change themselves, even rather young and small people. In order to change, a child has to first notice that a problem exists. He has to see what is. For this reason, helping children to see themselves and their predicaments more honestly is one of our prime functions as therapists. We do this in a number of ways.

"I put out the fire and pulled the alarm. If it weren't for me, everything would have burned down. They should give me a medal or reward," 13-year-old Dennis declared. "They really should."

Dennis spoke of his bravery loudly, but his quieter twitching and reluctance to look at me told me otherwise. Only after some 48 minutes of crowing, and my simply listening, did he admit to having accidentally lit a brush fire. By not putting him on the defensive immediately, his conscience led him to confess his crime. Once he could describe and see his situation for what it was, he was able to explore his occasional recklessness, poor judgment, and difficulty owning his misdeeds.

Much of therapists' intervening is to help children look in the mirror with the lights on and their eyes open. "What makes it so hard to tell me what happened?" I may ask a child, knowing the reasons carry more significance than do the facts of what's transpired. "You always say good, fine, no problem when I ask about school," I note to another, my noncritical words suggesting that perhaps any other answer is intolerable. To a third, "You say you hate being so mean, but you spent every minute of the hour humiliating your sister in front of me." By gently confronting, I try to encourage my child patients to see it like it is and to see themselves as they are.[7]

By maintaining a neutral stance not toward the young girl but toward her conflicts, we enable her to examine all the angles. For example, if she speaks of her need to do the right thing, I may wonder about her temptation to do wrong. In one case, I asked myself out loud why a child protested so vigorously the dangers of taking acid. I learned that her noisy statement betrayed her concealed and conflicted plan to try acid at a concert that weekend, a plan she decided to abandon. A more pointed assault would have sent her hidden agenda and ideas about drugs farther underground.

Much of our work intends to bring about insight. Although psychoanalytic schools propose varied and complex definitions, I agree with *Merriam-Webster's Collegiate Dictionary* (1993): insight is "the power or act of seeing into a situation" [or oneself—*me*].

> "I'm evil. Pure evil." Adam spent the first of his hours working hard to convince me that he was utterly rotten, berating me and everyone else with foul and demeaning language. "I don't care about nobody and nothing," he said more than once.
>
> But this teenager gave himself away in the twelfth hour. After cruelly celebrating a dead dog on the street, he suddenly interrupted himself to ask whether it might have been my dog. My noting his obvious concern led to a crashing down of his gangster persona, and his coming to note that, not only did he care, but that his caring made him feel exquisitely vulnerable to harm and disappointment. He came to see that he was much more a good boy than a bad one.

We often raise insight by bringing what is unconscious to awareness. When one teenaged tomboy came to recognize her deeply buried fantasies of marrying her father and her guilt over wanting to outcompete her beloved mother, she transformed into a feminine and confident young woman who could identify with both parents. Conversely, recognizing his occasional wish to be a girl allowed a heterosexual high school student to pursue drama studies, a creative interest he'd abandoned out of homophobia.

In these instances, I found that specific fantasy could wield obstructive power. At other times, we help our child patients to remember what's been repressed.

Curtiss was a bright boy, who was having serious troubles in junior high school. He felt constantly preoccupied, though he didn't know why. "I don't know what it is," he explained, sincerely perplexed. His self-consciousness led him to skip school, particularly to avoid school activities that involved exposure. He was unable to speak in class, let alone give an oral report. And being near girls was the worst. He worried that he might commit a sex crime or pee in his pants.

Curtiss's cure came quickly enough, After he'd gone with his mother to pick up his little cousin from preschool. Curtiss found himself about to pass out while passing the classroom's bathroom door. In therapy, describing that sensation led to his spontaneously recalling having wet himself in kindergarten while waiting for his teacher to get out of the bathroom. Of course, a majority of unrepressed traumata do much more damage and require much more therapeutic working through.

Likewise, we can evoke insight by reuniting distress with its original source. Children who can't tolerate the pain of losses and tragedies—or smaller narcissistic injuries—are prone to experience their distress in undeserving, confusing, and obstructing places. I've seen children whose sudden deterioration in school was caused by unexpressed fears that their parents would divorce. Once we put their fears in the open, these children could do something about it. Some children questioned their parents and learned that their fears were unfounded. Others discovered that divorce was imminent and could take action to better understand and cope with the sad reality.

Insight can come when children understand how they manage their life and its stress. "I withdraw from classmates not, as I've believed, because they're beneath me but because I fear my loving them and their leaving me." "I endlessly and compulsively line up my things not because I value neatness but because it soothes my ever-present sense of doom." "I brag not because I am so great but actually because most of the time I feel quite small and insignificant." "My promiscuous interest in sex does not attest to my maturity and appeal as much as it reflects my need for attention and something to help glue together my fragmented self."

Few children, of course, will speak these words. But over time—and with our support and respect for the important adaptive and protective functions these self-deceits serve—our patients often speak words that mean the same, their insights leading to more genuine ways of being and more openness to the therapeutic process.

In particularly intense therapies that run longer, transferential reactions, in which the child experiences the therapist as somehow being like a significant person from life outside of therapy, can facilitate insight.

My work with José had gone splendidly. He ran to the office, seeing me as someone he could admire and as someone to admire him back. Within two months much of his disruptive behavior had vanished. However, his migraines had grown more frequent and severe. This discouraging phase was accompanied by a dramatic shift in our relationship. José began to see me as unreliable and judgmental. He called me a bum and a loser. He began to experience me as colossally critical. He heard my softest sigh as a sign of boredom, my benign questions as frontal attacks, and our meeting only once weekly as indisputable proof that I wished to see him as little as possible and that I hated him.

Over many sessions, his certainty that I disliked him grew to the point where he tried to avoid his sessions. He pleaded with his mother not to make him come into the office. "Do you know what it's like to be with someone who hates you?" he screamed inches from my face. "Do you? Do you?" My comment that I was certain *he did* brought a flood of tears and the acknowledgment that his alcoholic and abusive now-deceased father had never said a kind word to José.

Too pained to remember his father more consciously, José began to paint a portrait with colors and shades of a man he knew much better than me. I became as awful as his father, with the difference, however, that he could confront me and we would work it out. When José expressed his rage in effigy to the man who deserved it, his migraines subsided. He grew more comfortable with good relationships with male adults and peers and no longer needed to see them as all good or all bad.

One doesn't need a full-blown transference reaction to use the therapist in this way. Children (and their parents) quite commonly come to therapy suffering harsh consciences. They readily project their self-criticism onto the therapist. "You don't like me." "You don't want me to get Hanukkah presents." "You agree with my mother and think I was wrong." "You're just like my principal." We help such children grow to live more freely and have more compassion for themselves by patiently demonstrating over much time that they are the ones condemning themselves.

For all our fancy terminology and deep theories, we as therapists help in other, simpler ways. We educate, showing our child patients how the world of people works and how they can have greater influence in that world. With our respect, honesty, and earnestness, we set an example that shows children how we conduct ourselves. We help them learn to be better problem solvers, clarifying their options and empowering them to make more effective choices in their own best interests. At times we employ behavioral methods too, encouraging their parents to build more structure into home life, for example, or by gently but steadily exposing these children to the situations that frighten them.

In the end, therapy helps mostly by supporting children's coping and living with their limitations and circumstances, enabling them to grow as fully and richly as possible. For some children, these limitations mean severe disabilities or horrid abuse. For others, it is no more or less than the basic challenge of growing up and human existence. Whatever our approaches or methods, our common goal is to heal what's been hurt, repair what can be fixed, and allow natural development to proceed. However sophisticated or impeccable our clinical work, it is largely our enduring interest, affection, and respect for the child's humanity and selfhood that carries much of the therapeutic power. Although love is hardly enough and the notion of the corrective emotional experience goes only so far, I am convinced that it is children's learning to truly, not narcissistically, love themselves that makes for the greatest progress, a transformation that can occur only with therapists who *really do like them* (Rogers, 1951).[8]

NOTES

1. Lenore Terr (2003) writes of a dramatic, terrifying, and effective 12-year-long treatment with a seemingly "feral" child who, as in her first year of life, was tortured and found beside her murdered 25-day-old sister. Although this case is unlike what most of us will deal with, Terr's conception of abreaction as an essential element of this child's healing can teach all of us. Even in brief and mild cases, shedding deep-seated distress—especially that which has long gone suppressed, repressed, or unexpressed—in the presence of a caring, safe, and empathic other (i.e., therapist) can be profoundly relieving and allow the child's self-exploring and mastery to proceed unstuck.

2. Nagelberg and Feldman (1953) discuss a case in which a child's withdrawal is a healthy attempt at insulation against overwhelming affective stimulation. See also my own detailed chronicling of an Asperger child's therapy (Bromfield, 1989, 2000).

3. For more detailed comparisons of psychodynamic and child-centered play therapy, as well as other approaches, readers are referred to Charles Schaefer's *Foundations of Play Therapy* (2003). While these schools differ, in my mind there's no question that to be a skilled psychodynamic child therapist, one must first be a skilled child-centered therapist. I also feel certain that a skilled therapist of either persuasion will be able to immeasurably help their young patients.

4. Readers are referred to Seinfeld (1993), especially pages 103 to 119, where he talks of Winnicott's conception of the *holding environment*. Think also of teddy bears and transitional experiences as it applies to a child's therapy and maturation en route to sound reality testing (Winnicott, 1975a). I send child therapists—and therapists of adults as well—to this British pediatrician turned analyst's writings (1974).

5. These concepts of mirroring, admiring, and empathy were pushed to the front of the stage by Heinz Kohut, a psychoanalyst associated with the Kohutian or self-psychology school of psychoanalysis. Kohut saw the basic drive of a child to be mirrored, taken joy in, and confirmed—all which help to cohere a secure and authentic self. Readers are referred to his original writing on the topic (Kohut, 1977) as well as a series of seminars he gave on how his work applied to child and adolescent psychotherapy (Kohut, 1987). For perhaps even clearer and more useful applications of his theory to child therapists, see Tolpin (1971) and especially Miller's (1996) guide to self-psychological child therapy. The more ambitious might wish to read Greenberg and Mitchell's (1983) challengingly dense classic on the evolution of object relations throughout psychoanalytic history. All clinicians are encouraged to read Fred Pine's (1988) seminal and significant article on the four personal psychologies: Freudian (drive-determined), ego, object relations, and self-psychology. Pine feels that there is truth to be found in all of the four perspectives and that each applies to every individual at different moments in space and time. His aim for synthesis has a lesson, too, perhaps for ways that the truths of the psychodynamic, cognitive, and behavioral may resonate or overlap.

6. That line of tension is the place where so much of everything happens in therapy. For a visual embodiment of this dynamic along with its many implications, particularly as they facilitate teens taking responsibility for their lives and treatment, see *Teens in Therapy: Making It Their Own* (Bromfield, 2005).

7. For a pragmatic look into the transference that can occur in child therapy, read Hannah Colm's chapter in Haworth (1964, pp. 242–256). Readers might also wish to learn more by and about the two "mothers" of child psychoanalysis, which means child psychodynamic psychotherapy. Anna Freud (1927, 1928), who wrote dozens of interesting and insightful

pieces on most every imaginable aspect of child therapy and development, was very much a traditionalist (an ego analyst) couched in the reality of everyday life (e.g., the family, schools, orphanages, hospitals). On the other hand, Melanie Klein, the *other* child analyst in the British psychoanalytic circle, proposed a much more provocative view of the child's inner worlds and ways to reach it. Although her dramatic conceptions—of oral aggression, infants' hatred, and primitive jealousy and envy—as well as her own aggressive brand of child therapy might startle some peoples' sensibilities, it's my view that she illuminates our work with children today. See Klein's own writing (1932) or Hannah Segal's able introduction to Klein's work (1964). Because these two women were so profoundly influential, readers might also wish to read about the "battle" between the Freudian and Kleinian child analysts (King & Steiner, 1991; Prado de Oliveira, 2001).

8. Carl Rogers (1951), the father of client-centered therapy, believed it was the therapist's *unconditional positive regard*, empathy, and genuineness that healed the client.

4

Do Fence Me In: The Bounds and Limits

Much of what takes place in psychotherapy occurs in the ether of human relationships, beyond our words and actions, in the recesses of our patients' and our own psyches, and everywhere between. It involves an ever-flowing interchange between two people in a more or less open atmosphere that can appear rather chaotic and defying of logic. But certain structures and reasons guide and ensure this sometimes glaring, sometimes subtle process.

THE FRAMEWORK

Consider a professional soccer game in which no rules apply. Players run in and out as they please, picking the ball up with their hands, passing it around like a basketball, kicking and tackling one another, ignoring the time-out whistles, lesser players deliberately hurting better ones or wildly climbing into the bleachers to beat on jeering spectators while equally outraged fans rush onto the field to assault the opposing team. Such anarchy makes for exciting television, but it would soon destroy the sport. Fans would avoid the stadium, and so would players. And as the level of play plummeted, interest in the sport would evaporate.

Although the overarching structure that oversees soccer seems stifling, the fact that there are stands for the fans, a well-demarcated field, and official rules for the players is exactly what permits the action to be robust, spontaneous, unpredictable, and genuine. Similarly, it is the sound and sturdy framework of therapy—framework being the dependable conditions and terms under which we meet with the patient—that guarantees safety and allows for the therapeutic process to evolve so freely, passionately, and productively.

The Space

Space is the first dimension of therapeutic reality. Its being well defined and enduring carries the most weight in a therapy.

> "Boingy, boingy, boingy. . . ." Circling the office, Raymond threw his body against every inch of wall. "Yup, they're okay." He opened and shut the windows. "In case a fire starts, but we probably have to worry more about burglars," he explained, tapping hard on the glass with his knuckles. "Strong enough." He did several heavy jumping jacks to see that the floor could hold us. Then, without a smile, he tried to slide his feet under the door as if to prove that he wouldn't fit. "If I want to leave, I guess I'll just have to open the door. And no one can sneak in either, unless they're a snake. Iiiiiii'm not crazy," he screamed until satisfied that the walls, windows, and overhead light hadn't cracked. "We're set for now," he announced, sounding unconvinced.

Raymond was a dangerously reckless and destructive child. He saw the office as a six-sided box like some cage, this perception grounded in his burgeoning delinquency and fantastic fears of being imprisoned in a dungeon. Unable to rely on his own skin and ego to keep his thoughts and impulses in check, Raymond had to check the walls, floor, and ceiling. He asked the right questions of therapy through his behavior. Can this office keep me safe from the outside world? Can this office keep the outside world safe from me? These worries took a shortcut to an even deeper concern: Can this office and therapist keep me safe from myself?

From hello to good-bye, the sturdy walls of therapy served Raymond and his therapy, enabling him to bring his more troubled self into the work and leading to greater ego strength and self-control.

Children learn quickly that what they say in my office can't be heard by their parents and siblings in the waiting room. Nor can what they do in the office be seen. Children appreciate that what they say can't be heard by friends, family, and teachers who are far from my office. This insulation permits children to open up more freely to me, themselves, and the therapy without having to fear hurting loved ones' feelings or retaliation for having spoken negatively.

For the less impulse-ridden child, the walls of therapy can define a space that becomes his own, even if only once a week. This enclosure makes clear that unless one of us flees, we—therapist and child—are stuck with each other. While this can burden the youngster who truly hates therapy or is going through a tough therapeutic phase, children routinely come to cherish our physical presence. After all, how often does a child get to "lock" himself and, for example, a parent in a room together to play and not to be disturbed for an hour?

The physical substance of the office contributes to the holding function of therapy. Children lean against the wall or slide to the floor in more regressed moments. In these highly vulnerable times, they rest easy, knowing that in here they will not be assaulted, stoned, or pummeled by anyone. Only when children sense a secure place can they expose themselves and their psychological underbellies.

That we meet with a child in a single room that's cut off from other rooms and the world conveys an important message: as long as we have you and me in the office, we have everything we need to do therapy—the implied corollary is that as long as we have you and me in here, we have everything we need to make a relationship. To do our work, we need no more than our mutual judgments and interactions. It makes sense that children who are particularly uncomfortable with feelings and people can initially find the therapy office confining and unnerving.

This discrete and discreet space physically gives children a home for their emotions and selves. Just as they skate at the rink, learn in school, and run wild on the playground, they come to associate being themselves with the therapy office. In a good-enough therapy, the closedness and closeness of the office increasingly takes on the properties of a (really big) diary or treasure chest, where children can bring their most prized and susceptible parts of themselves for safekeeping. Many children, especially those in turmoil, are instinctively drawn to the therapy office where their distress can be heard, explored, and put in its place.

For these reasons, I prefer to conduct therapy inside the office. Doing away with that therapeutic space, I fear, can sacrifice needed privacy and containment. Making the space in which we meet more open-ended can excuse the child from the anxiety-provoking closeness and growth-promoting relating that propels therapy. If a little girl can discharge her discomfort by kicking a rock as she skips or by running ahead, why would she ever stay put long enough to confront her issues and feelings? Is it a coincidence, I wonder, that child patients often request out-of-the-office field trips when they are most troubled, in trouble, or unmotivated that day to work in treatment? In some instances, going outside—for example, waiting in an ice cream store or walking through clinic hallways—simply wastes a good deal of our precious hour with the child.

On the other hand, there are more courageous, talented, and creative therapists than I when it comes to doing therapy outside the office. These clinicians know how to get children, especially teens, to do their work on the playground or on the way to a canteen or candy store. Although these clinicians sometimes go outside because there is no good space to use, their working outside or in an alternative framework more often represents a clinical decision that a teenager, for example, will find the office too close, too confining, too in his face. These therapists engage patients in their natural habitat. They shoot hoops and play tag, exploiting children's natural love for and inclination to connect around physical activity. In the end, it's a matter of therapist taste and ability. If loudly balking teenagers can grow to use and value the intimacy and focus of therapy in an office, so can they and their therapists learn to do therapy in the woods or while snacking at a picnic table.

The Time

What difference does it make whether we see a child for 10 minutes or 80, on Monday or every day, this week but not next? To begin with, there is nothing magical about the length of the therapy session. That it approximates an hour is a matter of convenience, practicality, and clinical experience. Sessions lasting hours would be overwhelming, hard to schedule, prohibitively costly, and completely unacceptable to insurance companies. On the other hand, sessions that are too short can make it hard for patients and therapists to settle in, and get to work. Doing 45 or 50 minutes rather than a full 60 is merely our pragmatic way to make room for note keeping, bathroom runs, phone calls, and a quick stretch.

And why once a week? A matter of convenience and practicality, this common arrangement is also clinically informed. Two or more sessions per week can make for a therapy that works faster and deeper, but two are generally more than parents and health care systems are willing to underwrite. Less frequently than weekly, however, can allow our patients to crust over, their psychic and protective shells growing back or hardening between meetings, making them less open to the therapeutic process and making each session feel much like the first.

Many clinicians see their child patients biweekly or monthly. Their reasons are many. To make the number of HMO-managed hours last longer. To accommodate parents' difficult schedules. To wind down a treatment, allowing the child to come less and less frequently and to grow more independent of the therapist. Some clinicians whose case-loads are too busy don't have time for weekly appointments, and others agree with some patients who say that coming less frequently gives them more to talk about. While there's no right answer, therapists' knowing the actual reasons for their decisions can help ensure treatment success, however much or little they and their patients meet.

The relative constancy of the hour also carries a lot of therapeutic weight.

Mario, an extraordinarily flat and near mute five-year-old, spent his first hour building domino towers. He said nothing when I warned him that we had five minutes to go. But he closely watched the clock for the remaining time. From that session on, Mario, who worked with his back to the clock, automatically stopped within a minute or two of the hour's end.

Mario's internal clock was unusually sharp. All patients, however, develop their own clocks. That regularity of time helps our patients to gauge their work. Patients bring up topics at the beginning, middle, or end of an hour. Knowing how much time remains enables children to prepare themselves for the end, for today's good-bye, so they may regroup themselves—their wishes, longings, and pains—before leaving the sanctuary of therapy to face life as it is. Like space, the time function contributes to our holding of patients. When a girl cries and cries at the hour's beginning, she knows she can "fall apart" for a good 40 minutes longer; another, with 10 minutes left, sees that she'd best summarize her tale if she really wants to get to the emotional punch line. A time frame also can facilitate issues related to separation and loss. Saying hello while knowing that good-bye comes in 44 minutes invokes apprehension of the end, a dread that tends to work its way toward the final minute. This measure pace allows the child to begin experiencing loss and related sentiments while still in the hour, while we are there to help her understand and work it through. We see evidence of this dynamic in most all of our patients, whether they rush out before we dismiss them or whether they dawdle, having to draw one more leaf or suddenly feeling a need to neaten our offices. "What are you going to do if I don't leave," one teen threatened, "call the police?"

In a similar spirit, scheduling our patients' hours acquires meaning beyond their merely coming to a time that we, they, and their parents agree on. While once-weekly therapy at any hour on any day is better than biweekly or no treatment, the sameness of appointment time accentuates its potency. That 5:00 P.M. on Thursday is *their* time evokes a natural process that resembles the inner spontaneous countdown from the start of an hour to its end. As children attach to the therapy process, they come to know and feel that today is the day or that the next hour is the hour. Children back from vacation will often describe with a sense of astonished curiosity their having thought of me while canoeing or playing baseball just at the time and day we regularly meet.

Having a time, day, and hour that is always theirs fosters children's sense of owning the treatment. While children can use therapy under the most erratic and vague circumstances, a majority seem sensitive to the conditions under which they meet. Even the child who is ambivalent about therapy appreciates that one real hour in the week, of the whole 168, belongs exclusively to him, is his alone to enjoy or detest, cooperate or fight with, value or trash. The steadying effect of a child's having an established weekly hour is convincing. Also, these constancies in time and space demonstrate more than our words can that we take this work and the child seriously. In themselves, they can be therapeutic for a child from a chaotic and unpredictable home, for instance, or an autistic child who craves orderliness. But it is our deviations from constancy that can lead to the real gold mine.

> Although I couldn't see him, Darren's loud sigh told me where he lay exhausted in the corner. For the past 40 minutes or so he'd worked furiously, using every conceivable object—blocks, game boards, tissue boxes, seat cushions, dollhouse—to erect himself an impressive, if motley, fortress. "Could you hand me the gun?" he asked, gathering up his last ounce of strength. He pushed the gun through a hole so that it faced the office door. "Now no one can get in."
>
> Not until he cleaned up did I learn the motive for Darren's hard work and upset. "You were with other children," he blurted out. "You like them better. Admit it!"

I'd been a few minutes late. But a few minutes was enough for Darren to notice. He saw in that void a reflection of his greatest fear, that his parents loved his sister more than him, worry that had come to permeate and obstruct his peer relations in school and on the playground. Darren's reaction to my seemingly negligible lateness led the way for months of useful work.

When our patients come to expect us to be on time, our being tardy takes on meaning. Just as parents nervously wonder why their children haven't returned from school, patients wonder what's going on. "Did I get the wrong day?" "Is he sick? Dead?" "Is he with patients he loves more? Perhaps he's mad because of what I told him last week." "Maybe he's masturbating in the bathroom (like I do). Or maybe he's smoking a joint in there (because, like me, he can't face life without a crutch)." The ways in which patients fill the black hole of our not being there are infinitely varied.

The prevailing scale of time is partly a function of our reliability. If we tend to be punctual, our patients may start to psychically rumble within minutes. If we routinely come late, our patients will probably react less intensely and after longer delays. While some flexibility can make our schedules easier to maintain and may appear to teach children to wait and be adaptable, I think it eliminates a realm of experience that, deeply reflecting the time-limited nature of life itself, is crucial to therapy.

Our ending on time is of equal interest. Do we let sessions run on and on because the child is talking, because he is almost finished with a skyscraper, or because he will throw an enraged tantrum should we stop him? No child likes to hear that "it is time," especially when having fun, in the middle of some meaningful play, or feeling the comfort of being with her therapist. As with beginnings, endings are also interpreted by children. "Did my therapist let me stay an extra 10 minutes because I was a good girl?" "Did she let me stay because she is afraid of my explosions and afraid that I'll make an even noisier scene in the waiting room and really screw up her day?" Or "How come she was so relaxed about my leaving last week but today she wants me out pronto? She must like me less this week."

I'm not suggesting that we live by those atomic clocks that don't lose even a second in a lifetime. I am instead praising the value of reasonable consistency, for without it we are left to measure what is happening in the relationship with a yardstick made of elastic. Moreover, unreliability in ourselves diminishes our right and incentive to recognize it in our patients. Clinicians who have trouble with punctuality are prone to dismiss that of their patients. How can we, in good conscience, confront a teenager's frequent lateness if we are equally tardy?

We expect children, which usually also means parents or other caretakers, to show up for their appointments. When a child misses frequently, we need to assess whether she's even in treatment. To ignore cancellations and no-shows can be self-deceiving and dangerous. We, the child, and his family need to recognize the situation and take action. I make clear from the onset that I will charge for missed sessions and last-minute cancellations. Of course, we do not charge for reasonable excuses, such as real illness, emergencies, problems, and so on. These terms are not to make me easy money; it gives parents a needed push when they are feeling tired, overwhelmed, or ambivalent about therapy. (I realize that some insurance, clinic, and public assistance policies do not allow clinicians to do this.)

When we commit to a child's therapy, we make an agreement to be there. If we cancel sessions at whim or a sniffle, how can we expect a child or parents to see our work as earnest? How can we tell Jane's parents that her suffering warrants treatment and then cancel her sessions willy-nilly?[1]

Limits

There aren't a whole lot of rules in relationship-based play and talk therapy. Although we hope that children will play and talk freely, the golden rule of analysis—to say whatever comes to mind—doesn't apply here so neatly. Sometimes we sit back and watch our patients follow their hearts and unconscious, playing at will and with ease until their internal conflicts and inhibitions get in the way. Children do not agree to therapy the way grown-ups sign on for analysis. In most instances, their therapies involve much more tangible involvement with their therapists. We do, however, as a rule ask that they be as honest as they can with themselves and us.

Because that's the shortest route to where we need to go, we follow our patients' leads as unobtrusively as we can, interfering only where we must. We wait and see, holding back our intervening until a child's actions or words call for it. Children, however, inevitably want to know what is expected of them. Struggling to define themselves in this context of ambiguity and competing demands (a task that looks a lot like growing up), they test us and the process like crazy.

Why don't we just tell them what's okay or what isn't or give them a handbook that lists the actions and language that are forbidden in the therapy room? To begin a relationship that way would convey a tone of authority and oppression that would not foster the open and accepting atmosphere we intend. Who wants to eat at a restaurant where the menu says "no talking with your mouth open," "spoons are to be used only for soup," or "no elbows on the table"? Furthermore, using the shotgun method to scatter a ton of prohibitive buckshot would make each child who enters our doors feel like every other child, likely offending children who would never attempt some or all of the forbidden behaviors on that list. Defining what can and can't happen up front robs children of the opportunity to make that discovery themselves, on their own terms and in their own time. Children tend to know pretty well what can and can't be done. Rather than impose premature structure, we set limits after the behavior or as it's occurring. But for that matter, why do we set limits at all?

For one thing, we can't allow children to hurt either themselves or their therapists. It's easy to grasp why a therapist can't permit child patients to hit him on the head. But even milder assaults are unacceptable. Allowing them implies that hitting and other aggressive behavior are good ways to express frustration. Hurting the therapist can lead a child to feel guilt or fear that the therapist will get her back—by hurting her or telling her parents.

When I entered the office, Bethany, as was her custom, jumped out from behind the door to surprise me, banging me in the face with an armful of toys, as she'd also done before.

I recognized that her exuberant greetings held affection as well as hostility, and I'd tried in vain to set earlier limits ("You can jump but not with toys in her arms"). Setting a limit on Bethany's entering the office before me became my only choice.

Although Bethany had not hurt me badly, the weekly whack on my nose and occasional poke in the eye were making me dislike her. My limit served less to protect me physically and more to protect my good feeling for her so that I might continue, as Ginott (1959) wrote, "to maintain [my] attitudes of acceptance, empathy and regard" for her (p. 161).

We also don't allow our child patients to harm themselves, though this can be a tricky path to hoe.

Victor had a long history of self-destructive behavior prior to therapy. Months into treatment, he felt more comfortable with me and had begun to show me his more anguished impulses to harm himself. I watched as he wrote hateful epitaphs on his forearms, occasionally pushing the pen hard enough to jab the skin. When the dull children's scissors failed to cut his bangs, he tugged the jammed scissors, pulling his hair out. When he stuck the point of an unbent paper clip up his nose and drew blood, I stopped him.

A reasonable reader may wonder why I waited so long? Consider Victor. According to his parents', his own, and previous therapists' reports, he'd mistreated himself for years and had twice tried to kill himself. Whether in mild self-mutilation or more indirectly with daredevil behavior and drug experimenting, he had long showed a wish to hurt himself. What were my choices? Like his earlier therapists, I could have hospitalized him. But to what purpose? That would have done little more than buy some time, putting off the clinical hardship we had to face. Alternatively, I could have refused to treat him whenever he did anything resembling self-injury. But I am not so full of my clinical self to believe that my withholding therapy would have inspired his self-control. Rather than corner him into healthier behavior, my provocation would likely have left him feeling abandoned and alone with his impulses.

And so, as therapists often do, I tried to accompany him down the narrow path that ran between self-caring and self-destruction. When Victor displayed behaviors on the edges of self-harm, I watched carefully and wondered aloud what was driving him at that moment. We'd usually find self-hatred. "I'm a piece of shit," he'd say, because he couldn't play a certain measure of a Jimi Hendrix song.

But when Victor took more hurtful actions, such as stabbing the inside of his nose, he grew less able and willing to verbalize what it meant. His clearer intent to hurt and not understand himself convinced me to set a limit. I refused to talk with him until he was ready to do some therapy. The positive leverage I'd accrued by my having stayed with him through a majority of his self-tweaking acts helped bring him back to me and the work. Victor put down the paper clip and talked. Limits helped me keep Victor just safe enough to learn what had fueled his extraordinary shame and self-hatred.

Children test us to gauge how much aggression we'll stand for. "Can we hit you?" (No.) "Can we push you against the wall?" (No.) "Can we spit in your coffee cup?" (No.) "Can we deliberately ruin your toys?" (No, though under some circumstances—for example, with a child who sadistically hurts others or one who's severely inhibited—I allow the torture of a specific toy to the point of its destruction.) "Can we attack your other patients as we leave the office?" (No.) "Can we shoot your Nerf blaster?" (Yes, that's why it's here.) "Can we shoot it at your face?" (No.) "How about at your butt?" (No.) "Can we at least shoot the side of your foot?" (No, because that's still part of me and you know it.) "Can we shoot my mother who's in the waiting room?" (No. While I generally leave parents to do their own disciplining in my presence, I do not allow my toy guns to be shot at other people.) "Can we shoot your pictures?" (Yes, because they are covered with unbreakable glass and the Nerf balls won't hurt them.) "Can we shoot your toy figures, your walls, your desk, your chair, and everything else in here that speaks of you?" (Yes, you can shoot anything that's not breakable.) Children's begging demands to shoot us testify to the strength of their wish that we respond to both their impulses and their craving for our limits.

In addition to keeping us, them, and the therapy safe, we have even better reasons to set limits on aggression that's aimed our way. By not letting children do whatever they might with us, we challenge their ego to contain the hostility, withstand the frustration, and delay gratification of the impulse. We let them know, however, that they can express their aggression verbally. Put it into words, we encourage them, knowing that they need the exercise of putting feelings into words more than they need to pound a human punching bag. By learning to control their aggression, here and there, bit by bit, children grow to manage it constructively and to verbally assert themselves.

I have no problem with children screaming at me, calling me this or that, teasing me, or sharing their fantasies of how they would torture me. Sticks and stones can break our bones; we know better about names. Most of the time, this behavior passes easily and clears the way for useful exploration of its meaning. Cases in which this putting me down doesn't let up, running for every minute of every hour, however, suggests to me that this purging of venom, while temporarily relieving, is therapeutically not doing much and should be checked.

Limits comparably apply to children's expressions of sexuality and affection. For the most part, children's fondness for us is generally a good thing. They make us gifts and heart-shaped "love you" cards. They lean against us when telling their stories and rest their foot on ours while drawing at the desk. Some give us hugs on their way in or out of the hour. What do these kind, sweet gestures have to do with limits?

Some children's wish to love us and be loved back grows excessive. They want hugs upon hugs and hugs that turn into kisses and more. Our giving patients that love would likely confuse them, for we meet not to physically love them but to do the talking and playing work of therapy. "Why," a child could wonder, "does my therapist hug me when I am sad but not when I am angry?" "Why am I getting love today but not in last week's session?" Our gratifying the wish for our love and consolation can detour the therapeutic process. While a frightened girl may want my arms around her, she will benefit more from my psychically holding her while we together try to understand her fear and sudden need for my protection.

Children's requests for affection often, if not always, relate to some psychological impetus. Children who incessantly and from day one shower me with love often do so not out of admiration but out of dread, their love meant to appease me and ward off the danger they perceive coming from adults or to feed what they may imagine to be my narcissism. Those children who plead for my affection are often riddled with insecurity about whether they are loved and lovable. In neither instance would my giving affection substantially solve their problems, soothe their longings, or resolve the larger underlying issue.

We must be particularly prudent about our physical closeness with children who have been sexually abused. Their trauma experiences may propel them to push for our physical affection. But our giving it would surely do more harm than good. Gently declining their appeals, we help them instead to understand why they so want us to love them that way: "Because I am frightened that sooner or later you are going to rape me anyway." "Because I only get love and attention at home when I act sexy." "Because that is what being loved by a daddy means to me."

Limits, while seeming to halt the child, can paradoxically move her ahead on her therapeutic mission. Consider a murderously rageful child who zings a paper plane at my face. What would happen if I should take a hands-off approach, say and do nothing in response? Seeing the plane jab my eye might shock a boy and evoke guilt that blocks his continuing to work on the anger he feels for a divorced and neglecting father who forgot his birthday. Excited by his hurting me, a second and less socialized boy might raise the ante, pelt me with dominoes, then markers, and finally large wooden blocks, until he brings the therapy to a dead end.

By setting a limit on a child's aggression toward me and diverting it to a more symbolic realm, the play and impulses beneath can go to their full and rich expression. "It's not okay to throw planes at me, but you can throw planes at this little me," I say, grabbing a play figure and setting it on the desk. In fact, that child will soon see that he can do virtually anything he wants to that plastic Dr. Bromfield. He can step on me, roll me in the mud, knock me down, drown me in a glass of water, put me in his pocket, or even kill and bury me. Setting a limit and redirecting the play into safer modes applies equally to matters of affection and sexuality. "You can't sleep with me, but you [or the plastic figure that is you] can do whatever you want with this Dr. Bromfield [figure]." On both fronts, the scenarios that children come up with are endless and take their play and thoughts to a more complete resolution than would physically using me as a real object of their hostility and desire.

Limits also serve to give our patients a needed place in therapy to express the childhood hurts that are too big and painful to bring up directly.

"That's it," I said, having stated clearly that drawing on the wall would not be tolerated. I put the markers in my desk drawer.

"You don't let me do anything," Anna screamed. "But you let everyone else do what they want! You don't care if the other kids draw on your walls. Only me," she went on through her angry tears. "I'm the only one you hate."

Naive bystanders—and many a parent—might think that Anna was overreacting to my not letting her draw on my wall. If that was all she was responding to, they would be right. But she was feeling much more. Her divorced mother had recently remarried, and Anna was justified in feeling left out. Her 56-year-old father had more interest in his own grandchildren, and her mother, infatuated with her new love, was much less available. "What about me?" Anna eventually confronted her mother and father. My limit gave Anna, who was originally unable to broach the topic herself, a hook on which to hang her resentment and a legitimate place to begin venting her broader distress.

Having established the power and necessity of limits, we should think about how to use them. They work best when administered matter-of-factly and with assurance, not when we are red with anger or at our wit's end. And they tend to work best when applied early, that is, when the child is better able to control herself. I do not wait to be hit on the head with a hammer. I set a limit when the child pokes my hand with a nail.

Whether we set a limit depends enormously on the nature of the individual child and the context. If a seriously well-behaved but inhibited child whips a hard candy at my head—a sign of his progress in treatment—I'd do nothing but help him to struggle with the guilt-laden aftermath of his act. However, when an impulsive child does the same, I'd set an immediate limit. If it continued, I'd end the session. Even when full of hostility, children who are attached to me and the therapy do not like being thrown out.

We try to set limits empathically. I know that, however clinically correct, stopping a child from hiding under my shirt will make her feel rejected by someone she loves and values dearly. And so, after I've set the limit, I stay open to the hurt and resentment I've caused. I note and accept the "I'm going to hate you back" that shows up in the talk and play that follows.

As with other interventions, the more judiciously we employ limits, the more effectively they work. We aspire to set limits that are in a child's best interest or that are in some way clinically necessary. Imposing limits sadistically or punitively or acting out some dislike of the child, anger at her parents, or frustration over her lack of progress will hurt the treatment. Some therapists shy away from limits; others run to them too eagerly. The best we can do is strive to know our own style of setting limits, paying close attention to when they work and when they don't, making sure to clean up any fallout they produce.[2]

Confidentiality

The issue of confidentiality is basic. While some clinicians suggest complex explanations and preparation, I think the surest way for children to grasp the matter is by our demonstrating it. Each hour that they share with us and each week that we don't betray that sharing persuades our child patients that we can keep the trust. This secure arrangement helps to hold the therapy and allies with the child's willingness to reveal and examine herself. Why would children talk to us if they knew we might just turn around and tell their parents?

Our preserving therapy safe from the outside world—isn't that essentially what confidentiality does?—also highlights for children our view that they run their own therapy, that they are responsible for its work. It stresses the need for their honesty. As long as we can rely on children's accounting of what goes on in their lives, the less we'll need to look to the outside for the truth. Confidentiality is an aspect of the honor system that exists between us and our child patients when we both keep our end of the therapeutic bargain.

I don't make a big deal of integrating data that comes from outside of therapy, mainly from parents and schools. I encourage parents to keep me informed and let children know that this two-way street of communication exists. I shy away from the CIA approach to informing. It is hard to make good use of information that comes from anonymous sources. If the school says that Arias is disrupting the class, I need to tell her how I know of this. That kind of secrecy seldom enhances therapy. Moreover, children will catch the drift that I and their parents or teachers are sneaking behind their backs, and that can jeopardize therapeutic trust.

As for parent updates, I describe what is going on thematically without giving away the specifics of the child's play or words. When I need to include the parents in something more pressing, I try always to speak first with the child, enlisting her help as to the best way to break the news. Sometimes I invite the parents in to the child's hour, sharing what I have to say in general terms, leaving child and parents to fill in the blanks. In those rare instances where I need to talk with the parents without the child's cooperation, I tell the child that I will be breaking confidentiality. My candidly spelling out my reasons for doing so usually leads to an acceptance and understanding that what I have done came out of caring and my best effort to do right by the child.

The matter of confidentiality raises the bigger question of the child therapist's ethics, a matter that acquires even greater significance in the contemporary context of shrinking insurance and health plan support for mental health services. After all, it's easy to do the right thing when the right thing is also the quickest, smoothest, and most well paying. Unfortunately, real-world clinical choices seldom look like that. *Ethics* means to do what we think is best and clinically right, even when doing so means clinically working harder, confronting more difficult situations or feelings, getting fewer rewards, or bucking popular opinion (including the parents' and school's). That we do most of our work in such an isolated and unstructured realm only adds import to the big and little decisions we make on behalf of our patients and their therapies.

NOTES

1. Readers are referred to Sandler, Kennedy, and Tyson (1980) for a highly readable and practical interview with Anna Freud. She explicitly talks of therapeutic space, time, and other meaningful essentials to doing child therapy.

2. Child therapists quickly learn the value of limits. Our child and teen patients—and their behaviors—force us to reckon with limits most every hour of every day. That is to say, you likely have already discovered much of what I tried to illustrate. Know that my own experience and views were informed by two classic sources on limits in therapy—the first an article by Hiam Ginott (1959) and the second a chapter on limiting aggression in therapy by Mary Haworth in the book she edited (1964).

5

Tell Me Where It Hurts: On Talking and Querying

Words are the currency of therapeutic exchange. While much takes place in the physical and psychic space between us and our patients, it is our and their words that most tell each other what is happening. What specific functions do our words serve, and how do we best apply them clinically?

Probably the most obvious function of what we say is to promote our learning more about the child. For some specific information, we simply ask direct questions. "How old are you?" "What grade are you in?" "Do you have any brothers or sisters?" Although such sharp queries can grow tiresome, they have their place in treatment. Beginning patients may appreciate a forewarning that we'll be asking a lot of questions early on but that we'll ask many fewer as we get to know each other better.

Closed-ended questions tend to elicit closed-ended answers—"no," "yeah," "3," "seventh grade," "never"—that tell little and put us in the position of having to ask a follow-up question, and another, and another, forcing us to make nags of ourselves. When we ask for pithy answers, we tend to get them, even from more cooperative and talkative children. In contrast, open-ended queries deter quick and easy answers. "Do you like school?" limits what a child can say and implies that any reply but yes is the wrong one. But "what's school like for you?" asks for all of the child's impressions, however big, small, many, positive, negative, or ambivalent.

According to one of the paradoxes that characterize human behavior, children tend to talk more to adults who ask less. And open-ended declarative statements seem to invite even more response than do open-ended questions. "You're at the new high school." "You've got a little sister." "It's a beautiful sunny day, and you had to come here." Children tend to respond to questions hidden in statements, as if they're most open to telling when they think we're least asking them to.

Questions typically arouse suspicion, causing us to wonder why someone wants to know and what they intend to do with this information. Guardedness leads to shorter, sparser, more defensive replies. Children frequently are so accustomed to parents' high-speed whats, whens, and whys that they readily note and appreciate our more respectful and minimally intrusive manner. They sense rightly that we mean our calmer query to stoke a discussion more than to collect evidence to indict them.

Of course, how we ask our questions influences the kinds of answers we get. "Oh, you're at Jefferson? You love it there, right? Doesn't everybody?" When we ask, do we allow enough time for the child to reply before going to our second question and our third? Well, if Andrea doesn't downright love that school, would she even bother telling us after all that? Peppering children with questions can make them feel attacked and give them the sense that we are mechanically going down a laundry list and don't really care what they answer.

How we react verbally to what children say contributes to how open an atmosphere we create. Do we make our child patients want to talk? When children tell us what they think and feel, do we respond with anger, criticism, or rejection? If so, we teach children to keep to themselves. Are we able to sit still and hear the whole story, or do we jump to conclusions and take panicked action?

Therapy is a self-exploration that requires patients to tell their stories. We try our best to let them do so as much as they can on their own. When they flounder, our urge to organize them is great, just as it is to complete their sentences or give them the words they can't find. Children will likely go along with us. But our interrupting implies that we have neither the patience nor the willingness to wait for them to talk for themselves. There's also a good chance that what we fill in is not what they would have said. When a child asks me where to start, I put her in charge. "Wherever you think you should," I patiently answer, certain that her choice will be best and revealing.

In the same spirit, I do not feign understanding, for example, laughing at a joke I do not get or showing sympathy when I can't see the hurt. I frequently ask children to explain a situation again or to repeat what I was unable to hear clearly. Should their reasoning fail me, I ask for their help. "I'm sorry. You're trying to help me see how your mom's birthday caused your fight at soccer practice. But I'm still not getting it. Can you try again?" When I admit my not getting it and acknowledge their efforts, most children are quite willing to persist. If they feel that we don't care enough to pursue them or that we blame them for our not understanding, they will often let the matter go and pull back a bit from therapy. Our overeagerness to oblige their "Never mind, it's no big deal" unwittingly says to them, "You're right. It's no big deal and certainly not worth any more of this effort."

Assuming that we want our child patients to understand us and we want to understand them, we strive to speak in ways to match their cognitive and development levels. Do we use words and syntax that they can understand? "You've experienced a great loss," while suiting an adolescent, would fly over most toddlers' heads and leave them alone with their feeling. Do we use 97-word sentences full of big words and psychological jargon that numb rather than touch our patients? Do we use complicated sentences, employing several if–then kinds of clauses or triple negatives that, instead of clarifying, tie a child's mind into knots? Is our logic too beyond or beneath the child's? Do we use irony or subtlety more fitting a literate and psychologically minded adult than a nine-year-old child with low average intelligence?

While experience and (clinical) practice tend to make us better at speaking to the child's level, we pay attention to the effects that our words have. Children's glazed expressions, complete changing of the subject, wholly unrelated responses, or more explicit "huhs?" and the like can tip us off that we are not making ourselves clear. Just as we persist in urging a child to get us to understand, we push ourselves to try again, asking the child where we lost him and making sure he knows that the problem communicating is ours.

What kind of language is acceptable in the therapy hour? For children, I think any they wish to use. After all, who knows better than they the words they need to express themselves? This doesn't mean we don't heed or probe the words they use. "What does that mean?" I have asked, with a smile, of a child who simply and defensively said that "school sucks." We could ask children to not swear, but to what end? To become another arm of the parental authority, confirming all their worst fears about therapy and us? We get far more by listening intently when they brave a longer and curseless phrase, rewarding them for that risk taking, implicitly encouraging them to talk like that more often.

I tend to curse little in the hour particularly with children who do so a lot. While sharing their street language may seem to be a good way of connecting, I wonder if I don't cheapen the therapy when I ally more with their protective, belittling stance against self-examination and growth. I have not met one adolescent who has found my "cleaner" language either offensive, distressing, or off-putting. They seem to pay me back, for the respect I show their language, with a respect for my own. I am more apt to curse with an inhibited child who struggles to make his frustrations and anger known because curse words can carry so much vitality when used sparingly.

Our language also is key in our establishing and maintaining an empathic attitude. How do we signal children that we are listening and that we know what they mean? We can reflect what they say to show that we grasp it. "You're so frustrated with math homework." "No one believes you." "Coming to therapy feels like punishment." Our verbal restating underlines for our patients what they've said. It shows them that we now know and gives them the opportunity to correct our perceptions or clarify what they meant. Speaking in this reflecting manner can feel quite awkward to beginning therapists, for few of us talk this way in normal conversation. When first attempting to do so, therapists may imagine their patients responding with "So, what? That's what I just said." And, if applied too often, too mechanically, and without true understanding, such remarks will strike patients as lame, robotic, and insincere. As with most interventions, our reflecting works best when used discreetly and at the proper moments, when we really want to confirm and emphasize an important thought or feeling.

We might also ask ourselves why we sometimes use extended psycho-babble to convey simple matters. Is it for our own or our patients' good? "You're feeling as if adults sometimes don't treat you with as much respect as you feel you deserve?" is a lot more tentative and circumspect than "You didn't like my asking your mother about your report card." The former and more distanced phrasing might well serve a fragile girl who can't tolerate a more direct stating of her upset with me; the latter might feel more empathic and real to a second girl who's more able to acknowledge her rage.

"That stinks." "What nonsense." "You're dying and I don't care." "You hate me and therapy." "What's the point of living?" Such short and pithy phrases, while sounding harsh out of context, can resonate acutely with the vivid feelings of our patients. Our caring efforts not to over-whelm them can lead us to weak speech that doesn't take an emotional stand and that leaves children feeling cold and alone.

Our discomfort with what the child says, especially about us, can deter our best attempts to empathize. Empathizing with a child's love for us ("You want me to have your flowers") is a lot easier than getting in touch with her pure hatred of and wish to destroy us ("You wish I was dead and gone"). Each of us has different vulnerabilities—involving aggression, sexuality, love, loss, or any other aspect of human experience—that we carry into our work as therapists. Our changing the subject or raising the level of discussion might, if we look, be an attempt to escape something that hurts, stresses, or repulses us. What really motivates our querying about homework when a girl talks of her smelly brown diarrhea? If we sidetrack her with our preferred interest, we will miss hers (in that case, a wish to smear my office walls with feces).

Sometimes we intend our interpreting to make what is unconscious conscious. Bringing conflict or hurt to awareness can allow children to see what is distressing them so—sometimes enabling them to make deci-sions about what they wish to do about it.

Lenny, a high school sophomore, was a good hockey player, but he could have been stellar. He was also a good piano student who his teacher felt had the talent to be exceptional. Despite superior apti-tude, he was a mediocre student in school, where he was exceedingly well liked by his teachers and peers. Although Lenny claimed that he liked how he was doing just fine and belittled his parents' and teach-ers' concern for him, he came to therapy willingly and dependably.

He frequently told of dreams in which he was unable to perform: given a test that was written in a language he didn't know, being unable to put the puck into an open goal, finding that his recital piano had no keys. He perpetually spoke with a longing admiration for those who achieved more than he did.

In about the fifth month of therapy, Lenny described a nightmare that had troubled him. In his dream, Lenny had been elected captain for his team's championship game and was about to be the hero. With seconds remaining, the score tied 0–0, Lenny was on a fast break toward the opposing goalie when the blades fell off his skates. Determined to overcome this mishap, Lenny kept skating until, inches from the goal and certain victory, he shot. The blade of his stick broke off, and the puck slid harmlessly to the boards. Lenny woke up in tears, not knowing how the game turned out.

"That's the story of my life," Lenny said with a regret I'd never heard him speak directly. Seeing that he continued to be distressed, I asked whether there was more to the dream. Lenny shook his head no. My gentle queries about various parts of the dream fell flat until I asked whether anyone had come to see him play. With a torrent of feeling and tears that blindsided him, Lenny recalled looking up from the ice, just before his skates disintegrated, to see his father's wheelchair rolling out of control down the Boston Garden's steep stairway. "Who gives a crap about a hockey game," he cried, "when your father's about to croak?"

A loving and good son, Lenny always had known how sad he was that his father had been paralyzed in a car accident. But he had never been able to see ways in which he was angry about having lost his father's physical involvement in his life. Nor had he recognized the guilt he felt about not being paralyzed, about being able to achieve and triumph beyond what his father could ever be able to do. By gaining awareness of his self-castrating way of coping—after all, wasn't it Lenny who held back his pursuits and who, in his dreams, would shoot himself in his own foot?—Lenny was able to grieve his father's injury. This freeing up, not so coincidentally, brought Lenny closer to his father and more able to see the ways in which his quite active father could still be a presence in his life. By coming to see what really bothered him, Lenny no longer needed to destroy himself or hold back in his life.

Although I do not do child analysis, I regularly find that repressed experiences and impulses can wreak havoc in children: hatred and sadism in inhibited children, yearnings for love and dependency in those who are habitually aggressive, homophobic dread in adolescents. Unearthing these can be as arduous and dirty as excavating buried treasure.

That some experiences are repressed and put out of consciousness is the most conspicuous testimony to their threatening vigor. The more potentially toxic to the psyche, the more deeply they're hidden. But we can't just cut them out, for they are not like cysts or tumors.

Clinical tradition, meaning the wisdom of experience, has taught us the need to respect the way children adapt to their stresses. "You're a frightened little boy with a tiny penis and no mommy." While expressing the psychological truth a 15-year-old near-delinquent boy feels inside, this observation would probably scare him from therapy. We instead work gradually toward the ultimate revelation. "You've got to be macho at Roosevelt," recognizing his tough-guy defense. "You can't let your guard down," recognizing his mistrust. "You don't need anyone but you," recognizing his inability to rely on others. And so we go, each comment peeling off a layer.

While quicker and more piercing interpretations can occasionally bring miraculous results, they generally go nowhere, or, worse, they send the child reeling. The most useful comments address unconscious material that is just a translucent layer below the surface. That is why remarks we make today can have so much more impact than similar remarks we made last year or even yesterday.

Because so much is unknown, mixed up, and not yet understood, our task is challenging. How do we comment or interpret in ways that tap what can be tapped, confirm what can be confirmed, console and confront, while reaching all levels of a conflict—doing all in a way that can be tolerated, grasped, and gainfully used by the child? The easiest way is by taking the time to consider *all* that the child says in an hour.

Alicia was frustrated beyond belief. Her parents always seemed to fault her. Her teachers picked on her. Her once beloved grandmother was turning on her. Her boyfriend was "a selfish pig." Her friends betrayed her. She had a headache. School was too hard. School was too easy. Her new shoes hurt. "Why," she asked me, "did you get such a bad haircut?" For pretty much the whole session, Alicia complained about everything and everybody in the world.

Alicia brought up dozens of issues that caught my interest, and I didn't probe any of them. I sat back and let her run her course. Rather than feeling the need to show meaning here, there, and everywhere,

I saved my interpretive arrow for the end. "Why doesn't anyone love me?" I asked in the first person. This rather simple comment brought a flood of tears and weeks of discussion about the ways she mistreated others.

What children express often reflects dynamics that operate on a larger and deeper scale. And so, we may strive to make comments that simultaneously access the superficial and deep. Consider a child who drew and then erased a stick figure of me, reflecting guilt-ridden conflict over a beloved uncle who'd molested her. My remarking, "You want to erase me away," confirmed the visible tip of a much larger and sinister iceberg. To have interpreted more directly her wish to kill her uncle would have overwhelmed her and reinforced her undeserved but nonetheless guilt-ridden conviction that the abuse was her fault.

Almost any therapy worth its salt would reveal a therapist and patient who've together developed a common language by which to communicate. Whether it is in the nuance, the rhythm, the specific words—be they typical, slang, or made-up—or the shared jokes, we create a cultural context unique to that therapy and child. For example, one boy early in his treatment ended a lengthy and belabored discussion of his wayward behavior by noting that sometimes he can just be a "rat's ass." For the remainder of his treatment, his exclaiming "rat's ass" became a short-hand signal that he'd screwed up and needed to fess up to what he'd done.

This evolution of a shared language serves two purposes. First, it allows us to share information, factual and emotional. Most child patients find talking to their therapist easier over time. Second, that language, known only to the two of us, therapist and child, acquires a specialness, propelling the therapeutic attachment while paralleling that between mother and child. Children prefer using this language to spelling out their complicated situations, thoughts, and feelings for they'd rather that we, like all powerful mothers, just know all that they feel and need without having to ask, without having to confront their separateness.[1]

Since speaking what is in their minds and hearts is a basic demand of their work with us, therapy constantly exercises children's capacity to put thoughts and feelings into words. Our limits further tell them that their impulse to action must be expressed in the form of play or, perhaps even better, in the form of language. And so, in the course of their therapy, many children grow more accustomed and better able to express themselves verbally. Instead of hitting, they can speak of their wish to hit; instead of cheating, they can speak of their wish to cheat; instead of withdrawing and rejecting, they can speak of their wish to withdraw and reject. For children who rely on their headaches and other bodily pains to speak for their conflicts, putting their feelings into words, particularly within an interpersonal relationship, can reduce the stressful toll their conflicts place on their bodies.

Our comments are also often intended to note discrepancies that our child patients are unaware of.

> "You say you don't need anybody, but you depend on your mother to do your homework, pack your backpack, get your clothes together, give you every penny you spend, and do almost everything else that other 16-year-olds do for themselves."
>
> Though Derek didn't like what I said, he recognized its validity just as he recognized my having waited many months to say it. Rather than argue my point piece by piece, week by week, and force him into a corner, I held on until Derek seemed close to seeing the contradiction between his behavior and words. I feared making him feel ridiculed or put down. What he heard was my observing that his weekly tirades concerning his utter self-sufficiency were self-deceptive. This contrast led him to begin a successful examining of why growing up frightened him.

Although it's tempting to hammer our patients on their heads with the contradictions we see in their beliefs and behaviors, such quick and heavy-handed tactics generally do little good and risk deterring the development of a strong working alliance. We tend to go faster by going slowly, by confronting gently and in due time. Rather than accuse Derek, "Who are you kidding? You're the biggest baby of them all!" I spoke in a more compassionate spirit that said, "I'm confused. You speak of independence and yet consistently seek its opposite. What does this profound and enduring irony mean for your life and how you live it?"[2]

This nonthreatening confrontation follows our relatively neutral attitude toward our patients' conflicts. When Kyle was terrified about water and his father wanted him to be a weekend sailor, I had to remain equidistant from both extremes. Otherwise, like his father, I would have been prone to push him toward the sea, or, conversely, I would have fueled his phobia, scaring him off from the sailing that he himself desired. As another example, when a boy tells me about his mistreating the family cat, I neither criticize nor endorse his actions. "Why does he *need to* hurt innocent animals?" is my burning question. The more open I am to both sides of the conflict, both sides of his ambivalence, the more that I and my child patient will learn about its meaning. Only when the child himself sees the reasons for what he does—"My mother loves that damn cat more than me"—will my hope that he treat his cat more humanely have an impact.

Whatever our patients' dilemmas—"Should I belittle my annoying sister?" "Should I disrupt the class?" "Should I forgive my unavailable father?" "Should I experiment sexually?" "Should I try out for the drama club?" "Should I go to that faraway private college or the local state school?"—we help most by inquiring about all possibilities, particularly those we disapprove of or can't understand. By doing so, we enable children to realize more clearly what they are thinking, feeling, and experiencing. We can push all we want, but only when Julie herself sees that she can be selfish to others and admits that she hates that about herself can we usefully take the next step to ask what she wants to do to be more giving.

Should a child claim that she *can't* [fill in the blank], I almost routinely reply, "You *can't* or you *won't?*" I've yet to meet one child who does not know the difference. True instances of *I can't* call for empathic support for children's helplessness and their predicament; those of *I won't*—including the cases in which a strong measure of won't mixes with can't—require more of a mutual press to know why not.

Just as talk is significant, so is silence. Those times when words do not come must be treated with the same respect and interest as those full of dialogue. What does a silence mean? Having told a long-winded or stressful tale, has a child run out of things to say or the energy to say them? Is that narcissistically fragile girl not talking because she saw us squelch a yawn, a sure sign to her that we are bored with her? Children sometimes don't talk out of shyness, embarrassment, fear of ridicule, anger, to be oppositional, and, most of all, because they may not want us or themselves to hear and know something about them.

Where does the silence come from? I am less struck by the silence of a child who is habitually a man of few words than that of a talkative child who, while telling of his mother's walking out on his father, suddenly falls mute. "*What is it?*" I am prone to ask a child whose quietness is seeming to be pregnant with meaning. When first hearing this question, children (and adults) nearly always have to ask what I mean and note the oddity of my words. However, after learning that I mean, "Why have you grown silent at this exact moment?"—and experiencing that as something legitimate to wonder about—that phrase becomes a powerful and useful tool for the remainder of the treatment.

My asking, "What is it?"—especially when posed in a period of obvious distress—often evokes tears and other forms of intense affect, underlining our need to leave room for silences to flourish and ripen. Patients will rush to fill in silences so as to avoid their discomfort and the revelations they bring; therapists often cut off silences, too, for similar reasons. Many conflicts and hurts require the stress and emptiness of a silence in which to bubble up. An extended silence, however, can be hard for therapists, stir up their own anguish, and tax them with feelings of helplessness and passivity.[3]

Being human, we continually have thoughts and feelings as we work with children. Many of these inner sensations tell us more about ourselves than our patients and are not to be shared aloud with them. Many others, while providing clues to the therapy, serve best by silently informing us and our interventions. As a general rule, by trying to speak only when we have something useful or helpful to say, not when we are anxious or pressured to talk, we preserve the power of our voice for the times we do talk and ensure that we leave plenty of room for the child's reflecting, feeling, and being alone with us.[4]

NOTES

1. For a detailed look as to how this would play out in a therapy full of idiosyncratic play and reference with a high-functioning autistic child, see Bromfield (1989, 2000). As you might predict, I believe that *every therapy* involves a perspective uniquely constructed by and personally meaningful to the individual child.

2. For the child-centered view of interpretation, see Ginott (1968).

3. Silence is a critical aspect of most therapies. Lanyado (2004) writes of her work with trauma victims, stressing the importance of the therapist's presence through the large and many moments of silence, and Harris (2004) chronicles a case study in which silence constructively predominated. I also recommend readers to the psychoanalyst Anthony Storr's (1988) reflective essay on solitude and aloneness, reminding us of their positive values.

4. Working intensely with children can stir up much that is deep and unconscious in the child therapist, and so aptly much is written about countertransference reactions in the child therapist. As an introduction, consider these writings dealing with rescue fantasies (Malawista, 2004), countertransference in residential treatment (Ekstein, Wallerstein, & Mandelbaum, 1992), countertransference working with disabled and ill children (Sutton, 1991), and working creatively with countertransference (Berke, Navaratnem, & Schonfield, 2006).

Part II

Techniques and Tools

6

The Lowdown on High Drama: Playing with Puppets and Action Figures

Puppet play can be fun, and the attentions of a responsive adult can be pleasurable. However, as is true for play therapy in general, the major purpose of puppet play is not to entertain the child or the therapist. Puppet play is nothing more than a vehicle to expedite the attaining of treatment goals, be they changed behaviors, symptom relief, self-understanding, or the freedom to be who one is. Puppets and action figures, found in almost every playroom, are frequently taken for granted. What purposes do they serve? And how can we help our child patients use them to therapeutic advantage?

Arguably, of all their many and important functions, dolls and action figures—the latter essentially being dolls for boys—serve to place conflict and other unwanted psychic stuff outside the child. Such exteriorizing is the most natural of human activities in the same way that we are apt to blame others when we mess up or can't find the keys or as seen in how easily we see our faults in others. While a lifetime of such disavowal makes for troubled and trouble-causing individuals, such externalizing within the context of therapy is an understandable defense against impulses, experiences, and truths that hurt too much to take on as one's own.

Puppets allow the child to safely express feelings that are meant for or were originally connected to real people, be they others or themselves. This displacing helps to ensure physical and psychological safety, which invites greater self-expression.

> "Here, have some more. Come on, you love it, don't you! Have some more." Jenna, an extraordinarily reserved and compliant seven-year-old referred for severe headaches with no apparent physical cause, cruelly rammed the plastic bottle into the small dog puppet's mouth. "There you go," Jenna continued, pushing the plastic nipple so hard she hurt her hand inside the puppet. "Drink all your vodka. That's a good baby."

Jenna was furious over years of neglect by her alcoholic mother. In play, she did to the puppet what she could not do to her mother. She couldn't even say these things at home for fear that her mother would retaliate or, worse, that she'd hurt her mother's feelings. Our shared perception that Jenna's puppet play, however earnest, was make-believe encouraged her to reveal feelings and impulses whose threatening reality was only too well known to her. In subsequent weeks she was able to tell, in direct words, how mistreated and helpless she felt and how she could not share those feelings with a mother she knew to be too fragile to hear them. Although magical thinking still led Jenna to imagine that her play might lead to more real-world neglect, that somehow her mother would know what she'd been playing, Jenna knew she'd never be assaulted or abandoned by the puppets, however badly she treated them.

Children can project feelings onto a puppet or doll, feelings they cannot bear owning themselves.

> "And those aren't crocodile tears, either." Eleven-year-old Jermaine heaved with drama as he made my alligator puppet cry.
>
> "What's the matter?" I asked the puppet.
>
> The puppet being too upset to talk, Jermaine explained that the crocodile's grandfather had gotten killed in a boating accident. "Oh," I soberly replied as I watched Jermaine comfort the puppet.
>
> "That's okay," Jermaine said, holding the alligator. "You'll be okay, fella."

Jermaine was a streetwise boy with an attitude. Whatever he felt inside, he wasn't about to show it. "Crying's for babies," he told me later, though he made clear that this alligator was no baby and had good reason to be sad. So did Jermaine, who'd lost his grandfather in a car crash, a grandfather who was more like a father. By putting his grief onto the puppet alligator, Jermaine changed it to a form he could bear and have compassion toward, thus allowing him to begin his mourning, a process that eventually led to more undisguised and heartfelt sadness.

But projected feelings don't have to be sad.

"Look at that stupid fag!" Thomas sneered. He'd deliberately squeezed a warrior action figure into a checkered dress that he'd grabbed off a small doll. He then topped off the outfit with a wig he'd made out of clay. "You dumb girl fag." Thomas took the tiny play scalpel from a doctor's office set and stuck it between the warrior's legs. "Now we'll cut it off and you'll really be a girl." The transformation complete, Thomas threw the warrior back into the toy bin. "You queer piece of crap."

By providing psychological cover, the doll allowed Thomas to share something that made him vulnerable to enormous shame. I did not wonder aloud whether it was Thomas, not the warrior, who really wanted to be a girl. My doing so would have ruined everything, short-circuiting the self-protection that this doll play was affording the early adolescent. Although Thomas discarded the she-warrior with utter disdain, disdain meant for himself, he listened with great interest to my empathic statement that life must be very disappointing and frustrating for a warrior who sometimes would rather be a girl.

Children prefer to see puppets, not themselves, as frightened, angry, worried, wanting. The puppet, not she, is the greedy one who wants it all. Or it's the puppet, not I, who wants my baby brother dead and gone from my house. By attributing their "bad" thoughts to the puppet, children transfer their internal conflict between good and evil to an arena in which they can battle the badness from without, developmentally, a much easier struggle. Unable to tell of her wish to be naughty, a girl played a fiery dragon who preys on a village. Somewhat the converse, I have seen a jaded and delinquent teenager turn a shark puppet into the God of the Ocean's helper, expressing in this play a wish to be a good boy, a basic wish that he forever disowned in his day-to-day tough-guy existence.

Children can project aspects of themselves that they just don't like. "Look at the fat slob," an overweight boy said of my unremarkable average-looking moose puppet. "You're so short I think I'll just step on you," another child said about the same puppet, height being that child's issue. My puppets have been seen as stupid, ugly, gross, deformed, klutzy, brainy, smelly, and having the wrong color hair or eyes. Sometimes what a child projects perfectly matches the reality, as when a child with Down syndrome, a child who was much teased for perpetually farting, tormented a plastic skunk for being so stinky. More frequently, children will see what they have to see regardless of what really is, such as when a girl who disliked her legs found my puppets to be "short and stubby," though of course she knew the puppet, having a hand hole in its bottom, had no limbs of its own. These harmless assaults, a spilling over of their own self-criticism, often lead to more compassionate acceptance of themselves.

All of these enormously varied self-representative functions can reveal much about the child. More disturbed children who lack an integrated self may employ many different puppets, each holding a limited fragment of their whole self. One autistic boy relied on an epic cast of characters, including the hungry wolf, cuddly lamb, angry moose, and sad duck. When feeling more intact, he would literally embrace all the puppets, feeling at one with them all (Bromfield, 1989). More advanced self-growth might be demonstrated as split or dual attributions, depicting good versus evil, needy versus satisfied, dependent versus self-sufficient, male versus female. In such play the puppet on the child's right hand might debate the puppet on the left, whereas better-integrated children frequently depend on one puppet as they confront and master their ambivalence.

As we've all seen, children often use puppets to play out interpersonal conflicts, especially those involving their families. Because these people, such as their mother or father, are absent from the playroom, the puppets serve as real objects to stage complex or painful situations. Puppets concretely enable physical action and nonverbal expression that speech alone cannot.

In our first meeting, six-year-old Jerry quickly stuck his wolf puppet in a dollhouse room. He used his other hand to squash several other puppets into the same space. Within seconds the police came and arrested everyone, except for Jerry's own character, the wolf, who now lay alone in the house, crying.

This was Jerry's visually telegraphic way of telling an impossible story of how his mother, her boyfriend, and various other lovers and addicts, all of whom frequented their small apartment, were busted by the police, leaving him to live with a relative he hardly knew. Readily available and easily manipulated, puppets empowered this overwhelmed child to efficiently reveal complicated events more quickly, succinctly, and richly than he could have with words alone, particularly in his first meeting with me. By widening his channel of communication, puppets gave Jerry a way to share his complex story without getting stuck or prematurely disrupted by the frustration of having too big a tale to tell.

Children's motivations for using puppets to act out interpersonal scenarios vary. Such play, especially if repetitive, may reflect a striving in the service of a developmental task, as when a toddler plays and replays a walrus puppet's migrating and return home. Analogously, children use puppet play to gain mastery over situations in which they've felt—and possibly still feel—helpless, frightened, or out of control. A recent kindergarten graduate orchestrated a puppet entering first grade. Another child, whose parents were divorcing, played a referee puppet futilely determined to make peace between athletes who waged colossal wars.

> Michael clumsily tried to make a larger lion puppet tie a knot with a string in its mouth. He explained that the puppet was securing the smaller lion to the back of a toy jeep. "He's not going anywhere." The bigger lion nonchalantly climbed into the jeep, then took off at breakneck speed with the baby lion dragging behind him screaming for mercy. "Yahoo!" the bigger lion celebrated, delighted by his cub's distress.

Michael's father was a roofer who'd make his son come along on jobs, forcing him to climb tall ladders and sit beside him on steep inclines. On weekends he'd take Michael for frightening joyrides on the back of his motorcycle. Puppet play provided Michael a safe arena in which to avenge his hurt, the play a springboard to our problem-solving ways to protect himself against his father's habitual and sadistic recklessness.

More simply, puppets can help a child to enact scenes showing what she has experienced or seen, perhaps to garner sympathy or support or to convince the therapist that her misdeed was really someone else's fault or that she was unfairly punished by some adult. Puppet play allows children, with relative safety, to tell *their story* replete with wishfulness, muted responsibility, and exaggerated heroism, often necessary and promising precursors to looking at themselves more realistically.

The manipulability of action figures and puppets perfectly suits children's need to turn passive experiences into active ones, reversing their misfortune into good fortune, re-creating circumstances to be less pained or problematic.

> Sandy tucked two plastic adult figures into the tissue box on the far windowsill. He then came back to line up seven little orange hats on the arm of the chair beside us. "These are how many lives we have." He then set up targets to shoot at, giving us each six missiles to fire. When we played and won—which he ensured we always would—Sandy made the two plastic adult figures pop up and run happily to where we sat.

Of those knowing Sandy's home life, who would not have been able to make sense of his play? He created a video game, the ultimate of control, in which our well-aimed aggression rewarded us with the return of a plastic man and woman. Sandy's mother was a scientist whose international reputation took her on frequent long and faraway business trips. His father traveled a good deal too, though not as much. "If only I could press a button and make my mom come home like that," Sandy later explained.

The fact that the child's hand actually sits inside the puppet also bears meaning. Like a facial mask, this hand costume can serve to create a sense of disguise, somewhat disinhibiting the child and fueling the "it's the puppet, not me" spirit of the play. The material limits of the puppet, its restraining the hand, can enhance the impulse-ridden child's capacity to maintain control while expressing potentially disorganizing material. The good feeling of the puppet's dark, warm interior can invoke regressive and sexual longings, stimulating fantasy play. And though the child holds the puppet on her hand, she may feel that the puppet *holds her*, a miniaturized and concrete embodying of the therapeutic "holding environment" (Winnicott, 1975a) that, in a small way, fosters feelings of psychological security.

Children use puppets in ways beyond their intended purpose as play characters. Puppets can be hugged, assaulted, abandoned (and retrieved), used as pillows, and folded up like a pair of socks to become a ball, to name a few possibilities. The fuzziness and softness of puppets can involve masturbatory urgings as well as provide less sexual self-soothing. Through these many and assorted roles, puppets can serve as transitional objects, helping children commute, in an increasingly realistic and mature way, between their inner experience and the world at large (Winnicott, 1975b).

Although neither necessary nor sufficient for therapeutic change, puppets can serve a helpful cathartic function. For example, the opportunity to shed real and mounting fears can buoy children facing painful and serious medical procedures such as cardiac surgery (Abbott, 1990) or bone marrow transplants (Linn, 1986). Beyond making the child feel better, emotional relief can lessen stress-related bodily symptoms, delinquent acting out, and other residue of overwhelming tension. A temporary discharge of anxiety can also make the child more accessible to education, reassurance, or problem solving that in turn can alleviate the source of distress or remedy a life dilemma.

Puppets can also help child patients manage their relationship with us, their therapists.

> "Will you feed me?" The Dalmatian puppet asked me in a small voice. Its master, a severely learning-disabled seventh-grade girl, handed me clay bones to insert in the dog's mouth. "Will you help me learn to do tricks?" it asked me, pushing its back into the palm of my hand. "Can I sleep at your feet?" the dog asked, making itself a snug bed on my desk.
>
> Allison gently removed the puppet from her hand. "Kids *really* play with these things?" she asked.

Puppets offered Allison a mode of communicating that allowed for physical activity even when sitting in a chair. The distance created by puppet play permitted her to test our relationship more vigorously. What impulses will we tolerate and to what intensity? What kind of language or silences are okay? A puppet can ask, perhaps months before a child can, whether it can have snacks, swear, or come as much as it wants.

While serving many of the same functions as puppets, action figures are particularly appealing to children who use them in every imaginable way. They can use them as family in the dollhouse. They can use them for target practice. They can put them into their beds, sit them at the kitchen table, wrap them up in tissue blankets, hide them, find them, throw them, send them sliding down slides into a father's waiting arms, send them down slides into a cauldron of boiling oil, wrap them up in cellophane-tape straitjackets, or even cram them into the dollhouse toilet. And they are just the right size to be eaten by my hollow rubber *Tyrannosaurus rex*. Their handy size makes them convenient, rough-and-ready stand-ins when children stage their therapeutic crimes and dramas.

Superhero figures are perfect to express omnipotent fantasies of unlimited powers and strength, particularly for children who feel weak and helpless bodily, psychologically, or circumstantially. Army men and military-type figures tend to evoke battles involving aggression, pitting good against evil. Civilian setups, such as action figure classrooms and doctor's offices, obviously work well for children playing out conflicts related to those settings.

The dollhouse itself is a useful vehicle for children's play in treatment. Whether portrayed as an impenetrable fortress against intruders and tornadoes or as a home of straw to be easily destroyed by the wolf's first and feeblest huffing, it teaches us much about the child's world. Our child patients can use the dollhouse to construct their homes as they are or as they wish they were (the latter, not uncommonly, resembling the homes they assume that we, their therapists, live in). Sometimes children set up the dollhouse mostly as a test to see what happens next week, to see whether I let other children mess it up. Their eventual discovery that I let every child use the dollhouse, however grandly set up by the child before, invariably summons issues of competition (for attention and love).

As with any aspect of play or talk therapy, the therapist must be willing to proceed at the child's pace. Even under the pressures of managed care, no patient can proceed faster than he can. The therapist intervenes, saying or doing something, only when there's something useful to say or do.

When a child's puppet addresses me, I try to respond directly to the puppet, making eye contact with it and talking to it. Children watch closely to see how genuinely we participate in the charade of puppet play. If we interact with the child, ignoring the inquiring or advancing puppet, we risk undoing the original motive for using puppets and undoing the therapeutic impetus. Just as we would not insist that a child play or talk, we do not make demands of the puppet. Rather than order the "barking Snuffy" to speak English, we might note that "Snuffy is barking," and only later and gently invite the puppet dog to share more, in words.

For many minutes we'd sat in silence, Gary and I making our identical skunk puppets stare into each other's eyes. We intensely watched our characters as if observing a real meeting of living and autonomous creatures.

"Why's he crying?" the third grader finally asked.

"I'm not sure," I answered.

"He's probably sad about something he can't talk about," Gary explained.

Since his mother had been diagnosed with breast cancer, the once cheery boy had grown sullen and was unable to work at school. He had severe stomachaches and slept poorly. But he hadn't shed a single tear and hadn't been able to share his worry with anyone. Allowing our puppets to quietly gaze at one another helped fuel Gary's perception of the skunk puppets as "sufficiently alive to give the illusion of a human being with whom one can speak, who will reply and who will actually move" (Rambert, 1949, p. 17). This small interaction opened the gates to Gary's improved coping with his mother's illness.

The emotional revelations of puppets cannot be hurried. Acceptance of emotions can be conveyed nonverbally, for example, by gently pushing a box of tissues toward a baby frog who cries. When a puppet looks a certain way but is not described to be feeling that way, I am wary of prematurely defining the affect. If a child crunches up a lion's face, we might first note that the "face is all crunched up" rather than "the lion is sad." If we guess wrong, we confound the child's own line of inquiry. Should we guess right, we run the risk of chasing the child away, repeating some parents' tendency to feel and act as if they know what's in a child's mind. What patients spontaneously offer usually proves more valuable than what we forcibly extract.

As a rule, children are willing to steer their puppet play. Exuberant therapists, especially those who pride themselves on their playfulness and access to fantasy, may be prone to overpowering the child, influencing the play's direction according to their own biases and needs. Contrary to what one might expect, a child typically does not mind being asked, "What should my alligator say [or do] now?" This query urges our child patients to lead the way, opening our window to their psyches and making our job as therapists easier.

Over sessions, we watch for continuity but allow for change. When a child wishes to name the puppets, preserving their names and qualities, our recall of that is appreciated and conveys deep caring. However, that child may one day wish to start anew, making fresh characters with previously unheard-of names. Should we run to show that child that his earlier play was remembered, we may inadvertently retard the natural evolution of play. In such a situation we might ask, "Do you wish to use new names?" or "Is the cow's name still going to be Mr. Bull?"

Some children grow quite invested in and attached to the puppets, using them to express deep and personal feelings. When a child removes her hand from a puppet, her caring may continue. I take care not to mistreat a puppet in the child's presence, for example, tossing it across the room into a toy box only moments after that same puppet has expressed heartfelt grief. The child, however, holds the right to mistreat the puppet that just seconds ago was her dearest confidant. That is the patient's prerogative.

All aspects of puppet play, including form and manifest and latent content, are fair game for our observing and examining. In every instance, we work together with the child to decipher the meaning and motivation of the play, keeping in mind that puppets and their acts often carry multiple meanings and motives. For example, a sadistic father puppet may reflect qualities of a toxic real parent as well as the child's own hostility. Wild analysis of puppet play, as of any other words or deeds, is of little value and can cause harm. By our showing the child's puppet acceptance, admiration, empathy, and judiciously reasoned interventions, the child comes to feel the same in kind.

While many children immediately take to the puppets, other children can be pushed toward them, as a form of limit setting, when perhaps their sexual or aggressive play is becoming too intense or dangerous.

> Keith, a first grader who'd been molested by a camp counselor, could not talk of the incident. However, in his third hour he became more vocal. "Kiss my belly." He lifted his T-shirt. "Feed me a banana in my butt. Do it. Do it!" As his voice grew louder, he also came closer, abruptly trying to stick his hand under my shirt.
>
> "Here you go," I said, standing up and handing him a puppet. "It's not okay to go into my clothes, but you can do whatever you wish with this guy." Keith eagerly took the puppet he designated to be me.

By suggesting that Keith use a puppet while making clear that his provocative behavior could not be targeted directly at me, I helped him to continue his play associations. This limit redirected his affect and deeds into symbolic play, enabled me to sustain an accepting and empathic posture, ensured our mutual safety, and strengthened his ego controls (Ginott, 1959). After all, I was not about to let Keith kill, maim, cook, eat, or rape me, but he could—and with great therapeutic benefit did— do those things (and more) to my puppet namesake.

By allowing a greater and safer opportunity for action of all kinds, puppet play helps children preserve their therapeutic themes and momentum. For similar reasons the puppets make wonderful companions to the doctor's kit, for so much of what my child physicians want to do to me is not allowable (e.g., where they want to stick the needle).

The special role that puppets play in child therapy derives mostly from their facilitating value, their expansion of the communicative repertoire between child and therapist. Through its many functions, puppet play both invites and enhances the intimacy, disclosure, and self-discovery essential to relationship-based therapies.[1]

NOTE

1. The material in this chapter was derived, in part, from "The Use of Puppets in Play Therapy" by R. Bromfield, in *Child and Adolescent Social Work Journal* 12(6): 435–444, copyright © 1995, and used by permission of Plenum Press.

7

Shoot, Topple, and Roll: Using Games, Building Toys, and Guns

---

While puppets and dolls most visibly seem to personify what children think and feel, they can use other play materials to show themselves and to manage being with us. How do children employ games, building toys, and play weapons in their therapies, and how can we maximize their self-clarifying functions?

GAMES

The love of games that the majority of children know does not wait outside the therapy office. "Great! You have Life." ". . . Chutes and Ladders." ". . . Uno." Just seeing their favorites on our shelves puts their minds a little more to rest as they reckon with their having to be in a room with these strangers doing whatever strange business we do. That we have such games tells them, so they assume, that we must like children and like games or at least understand and respect what *they like*.

More important, the games' presence suggests that we will be playing games, subduing some of the child's anxiety about how this apparently open-ended and free-flowing hour will be spent. But what do we actually do with games once the therapy is on its way, and how do they help to propel it?

The most obvious function of games is also the simplest. Games make children feel comfortable. The material substance of the game, the playing board or card piles, defines an occupied space that helps to organize the child's physical relationship with the therapist. I sit here, you sit there, and neither of us moves any closer. To varying degrees the structure of the game tells the child what to do: he needs to pick a card, read it, and move the game piece as the card dictates. The mechanics of the game—throwing the dice, spinning the pointer—demand attention, limiting how much a child and therapist can talk about personal matters. The overriding play of the game—my turn, your turn—repeatedly and dependably enables the child (and the child's therapeutic load) to be saved by the bell. Holding the cards or counting out the play money gives children something to do with their hands, helping to bind their anxiety.

Playing a game can draw out a child in all of these ways. In the absence of a push or demand to talk, a child may suddenly feel an urge. "My teacher's such a jerk," spoken incidentally while slamming down a winning gin rummy hand, can be the beginning of a constructive discussion of school-related issues. Insulated by the board, distracted by the playing, interrupted by turn taking, and expected to make eye contact with the game, not us, children can find themselves feeling more relaxed and secure. Much like the kibitzing-inducing powers of bridge or poker, the pleasures and camaraderie of playing games with us can lead children to surrender their guard and begin to reveal themselves.

But we must play our own therapeutic cards carefully. Should we blow a whistle, jump up and down, suddenly stop playing, or show too much attention to our child patients' toes-in-the-water revelations, we will send them scurrying back to their shells like so many startled hermit crabs. Thus, some turns later, I reply, "Your teacher's a real jerk?" My delayed response implies a lack of urgency, my eyes on the game, not him.

We must be wary of relying too much on the facilitating value of games. Some children, particularly those uncomfortable with the notion of sitting with a therapist, want to play games a lot, if not all the time. For these children board games such as Diplomacy, Risk, and chess reign supreme: by their figuring, the bigger the game (meaning more time consuming and more complicated), the smaller the burden of talking and being with us. Although these children may protest that they can play a game and talk, often they do little more than hide behind the pawns and knights.

For this reason more intensive board games might best be tucked away for special circumstances, as when working with a child who cannot tolerate therapy otherwise. To unnecessarily introduce therapy with these kinds of games can unintentionally trap the therapy, fostering the child's dependency on such a structured crutch, denying her the hour-by-hour experience of getting used to the talking and playing of therapy. In addition, therapists are prone to run to the games with patients to whom we feel unable to connect or with whom we feel lost as to what to do for the hour. Like the parents we counsel, we sometimes need to reassess our choices. It's okay—and perhaps necessary—for us to change our minds midtherapy, to decide to tell a child that we won't be playing Monopoly anymore, further explaining that when we do play it, we just don't seem to get the (therapeutic) work done. Even if the work is going forward, we are obliged to put the game away if we judge that it would go faster and better without the distraction.

For some children the social aspect of playing a game is constructive.

Randy loved playing Ladybug, a board game in which snails race a spiraling track to the prized ladybug. When first playing, Randy cared only about his turns, needing to be reminded to give me the dice and a chance. He routinely and unintentionally knocked my snail off the board as he moved his own. Randy might as well have been playing by himself.

But it was a good thing he was playing with a therapist, for his egocentric ways had cost him many friends. Even his mother and father didn't like playing with him. As he played the game over and over with me, we came to understand that much of what he did was no more and no less than his naturally unthinking and clumsy way. He had to work hard not to throw the dice everywhere or to move his snail without disturbing my own. My compassionately helping him to see this allowed Randy to begin making allowances for himself. He came to see that he couldn't help messing up the board sometimes, but he could take the time and effort to set it back up to where it was. Slowly he also came to see what it must be like for me to be constantly overlooked in the game. Without my telling him what to do and without group child therapy, Randy transferred his insights to become a better game player and playmate outside of treatment.

In a comparable fashion, playing games can help children come to terms with their learning disabilities. Although she enjoyed games and friends, 11-year-old Cheri's cognitive problems made game playing difficult at times. She routinely moved her playing piece the wrong number of spaces or even the wrong way, both to and against her advantage, and unwittingly broke the rules. More times than not, she miscounted play money and could not add her points in score-tallying games such as Yahtzee. In short, she loved games but could barely play them. The few she could play with some competency, such as Candy Land, bored her fellow sixth graders. Cheri's game playing typically ended in her quick and utter frustration, with playing pieces and game board thrown everywhere.

In her work with me, we repeatedly observed the little big things that called attention to her weaknesses and led to her self-hatred. "I'm so stupid. My cousin in kindergarten can play games better than me." Our work proceeded space by space, roll by roll, even more slowly than did our snail-playing pieces. Over time and many aborted games, Cheri came to see how her learning difficulties impaired her playing. She grew to have compassion for herself for having to work so hard at something that came so easily and pleasurably to other children. Rather than reflexively despise herself for being so stupid, she learned to laugh at herself and her inevitable mistakes. She developed coping strategies, for example, learning to banter comfortably while buying herself more time to ponder or make her move. She became more self-protecting, declining to play games that were too much for her and becoming a better negotiator with friends about what games to play. Being such a game lover, she decided to practice more, trying games on her own at home to prepare to play them with friends. Most of all, she came to better accept her limitations, not just when playing games but also at school and home, allowing her to make better use of the help that her parents and teachers offered.

Games that demand skills beyond the intellectual can similarly exercise children with issues around their perceptual-motor skills. A child's lack of skill at games requiring dexterity, such as ring tossing or dart throwing, can bring up feelings of incompetency and low self-esteem as well as raise even deeper issues involving, for example, one boy's belief that his father, an athlete, loved him less for not being one. This type of game can also help to inform us about how accurately our child patients assess their abilities. Is the child as inept as he moans he is, or is he actually better coordinated, his self-criticism reflecting unreasonably high standards?

For obvious reasons, game playing provides a forum to deal with conflicts around competition.

> An extremely bright child, Joshua would play cribbage keenly and to the death until it appeared that I would lose, at which point he became a bumbling and inept rival. Afraid of winning but not wanting to lose either, Joshua most liked hard-fought ties, those circumstances in which he could play tough without suffering the guilt of victory. When unable to avoid winning, Joshua would make endless excuses on my behalf, dismissing his triumph as lucky and meaningless. My noting his having won fairly and deservedly led to his solicitous appeals out of worry that I might be angry and resentful of having been shown up.

Joshua's oedipal conflicts—meaning in this case his fear that beating his father would result in loss of his love—led to his profound under-achieving not only in games but in most areas of his life. As we continually noted his conflicts around our competing, he came to understand his fear of winning. Progress in the real world accompanied these insights. He became more assertive in expressing his ideas and creativity and more able to compete intellectually in situations that allowed it (e.g., spelling bees and debating club). Joshua engaged in several new activities, such as athletics, that he'd previously avoided. He also came to have an easier and more satisfying relationship with his father, who Joshua had assumed incorrectly couldn't handle his maturing and growing competencies. Above all, he grew capable of feeling the pride and joy of his many accomplishments and was willing to try things he was not quite so good at.

Games can prove highly relevant to the therapies of narcissistically vulnerable children for whom losing is a dreaded injury to be avoided at all costs.

> "Come on, you bastard. Deal the cards. What a piece of crap you are. You can't even shuffle cards good," Fritz accused.

These tirades were no surprise. When I won at pick-up sticks, he accused me of cheating. I'd also, so he judged, tricked him at Chinese checkers. The sorest of losers, Fritz was not even a pleasant winner. "Loser. You're such a pathetic loser. I can't believe how stupid you are."

By our struggling around each and every game and by examining his need to put me down mercilessly, Fritz grew stronger and more able to withstand the outcome of the game, whether he won or not.

"Why, when you win, do I have to be a complete fool?" "Why, when I win, do you need to believe that I won by dishonesty?" "Why can't we both try hard at a game in which only one person can win? And for that matter," we came to ask together, "why can't one of us win without either of us being worthless or sleazy?"

Rather than try to teach Fritz to play fairly, I provided a safe place for him to recognize just how badly he had to win. Rather than criticize his ruthless game playing, I respected his need to protect an utterly fragile self-image that losing a game of checkers sent reeling. By the time Fritz could say out loud (and with a smile), "I must win every game!" he'd grown tolerant of losing and sometimes even intentionally misplayed to let me win. The insights of our game playing eventually led to our dealing with his bigger susceptibility to narcissistic injury from the world in his life outside of therapy.

Playing with children like Fritz forces therapists to confront the question of cheating. With Fritz, for whom winning meant surviving, I chose not to confront or limit his cheating. To do so would have put him on the defensive and neglected the all-important protective function it served. As he became more aware of that need, he himself began to note, with laughter and delight, how sneaky he could be. He gradually gave up his cheating. His playing pieces would act out his sentiments by teasing my piece, knocking it down, and literally running rings around it, bringing his once deceitful cheating into the therapeutic realm for examination. However, as with most matters of therapy, there are no golden rules we rely on when a child cheats.

We try to assume that children who cheat for either our benefit or their own are conflicted. When they flaunt their cheating in our face, it suggests they are acting out something interpersonal, wanting our attention, our reaction, our limits. In those instances, our noting their amusement and following where it leads will suffice to explore what it means and lead to the child's giving up the behavior. Often we find that children who cheat in this way are telling us that they feel one down or in some way impotent in their world and needing extra power to their advantage.

But when we work with more singularly sociopathic children, those lacking consciences or who teeter on the fence between decency and delinquency, we may not wish to humor their cheating, especially when intended to manipulate us and the game without our knowing. "You moved your man an extra space," I do not hesitate to point out, wondering out loud why he needs to cheat. "Cheat much?" I'll ask, listening carefully to the bragging list of ways in which the child beats the system and his playmates. While our discussion and game playing may help, it is a steady combination of empathy and limits, with heavy behavioral intervention in his school and home life, that promise the most hope and help to the seriously wayward child.

The game playing itself can carry a symbolic meaning for the child. One high school senior, anticipating college, found herself drawn to Candy Land, which evoked intense memories of a childhood and home she was unsure about leaving. Its opposite is the overcoddled first grader who brought a chess set to his session, proclaiming that my games were for babies. Young children use through-the-forest-type board games to play out fears of a dangerous world and growing up. Games such as Sorry and Chutes and Ladders give our patients a wonderful opportunity to safely express their aggression as they gleefully send us back to Go or watch us slide backwards to square one.

The framework of the games we play also tends to bring up much for the child. The child's view of questions concerning who goes first, who's the banker, what constitutes winning, and who, winner or loser, starts the next game become fodder for examining. And what do we do when the hour ends but the game isn't done? If it's a child whom life is forever stacked against, I might let her finish her triumph unless she's losing, in which case I might stop and spare her the loss. A child and I may decide to record where the pieces are and whose turn it is so that we can resume the game next hour. With a child for whom feeling loved and being loved are issues, I might go a little longer, symbolically giving extra. Then again, for a child provocatively squeezing a 20-minute game into the remaining one minute, I might opt to end the game and session on time. *It all depends.*[1]

BUILDING TOYS

Thirty-two large cardboard blocks are the most used toys in my office. I suspect their popularity is attributable to their value in so many varying kinds of play. Being large and easy to hold, blocks make a rough-and-ready toy that especially suits younger children and those with motor difficulties.

Blocks offer the child an easy way to be with us in the beginning, a way that allows for physical movement and fairly certain success. Many children initially use them to build towers, seeing how high they can go, taking great pleasure when their blocks pass my head or reach the ceiling. These constructions early in therapy, I've found, often move the child to ask that we invite their mother or father in from the waiting room to show off their creations.

In a simple and concrete way, blocks enable the child to work on a problem, such as making a tower that won't tumble. Through repeated trial and error, children can experiment their way to a stronger and taller structure, each bit of success enhancing their confidence and giving them a greater sense of influence over their environment and world. It is impressive, indeed, to observe children push themselves to higher standards and more complex designs as they progress, making clear that it is the process, not some static result, that motivates their efforts.

Children use blocks to facilitate their fantasy play with other toys, building zoos for their animals, garages for their cars, and homes for the puppets. One 12-year-old used such a setup to resolve his dislike for a new stepfather.

"We only have a couple of minutes left," I announced. "Just one more thing," Devon replied as he put the finishing touches on an elaborate army base he'd made out of blocks, the base's invincibility apparently uncertain. Devon had placed a green army man, gun, or tank in every nook and cranny of his construction. "There," Devon said. He placed one lone soldier to face that formidable force. "That's your army." Devon spent the last seconds demolishing my one-man battalion.

For months, Devon replicated this play, each hour giving me a few more men, then some guns, then tanks. Although he never once mentioned the stepfather whom, I knew from his parents, he resented for having stolen his mother and for trying to enforce rules like a real father.

Devon's relationship with his stepfather steadily improved. By the time our forces equaled out, Devon was able to describe how small and overpowered he felt by his parents' divorce and his mother's remarriage. By maintaining the security of his sturdy block base, Devon was able to relinquish and share more of the power with me and his stepfather.

Children soon realize that the same blocks that can be used with puppets and action figures can be used to build things big enough to accommodate their own bodies.

> Eight-year-old Coby was an impulsive and anxious boy who couldn't sit still. The fact that he'd recently suffered a first epileptic seizure heightened his fear of losing control. For months Coby lay on the floor while I built block walls around him, walls he'd suddenly break through with kicking and thrashing. Each week he asked that the bordering blocks be brought closer to him, requiring that he lie increasingly motionless so as not to disrupt them.

By controlling his body to be perfectly still, then cataclysmically wild, Coby began to master his self-control as well as his dread of another seizure. This mastery brought increased coping with his illness, a willingness to learn techniques to relax, more cooperation with his medicine, and more constructive expression of the rage he felt over having epilepsy.

Children frequently build block fortresses and walls to hide behind, protect themselves, and shut us out. "My mother can make me come here, but she can't make me talk to you," one ambivalent child called to me from inside the cave he'd built himself. He was right, too. The shelter of his cave, however, allowed him to engage with me around his misgiving about therapy, a connection that soon brought a strong attachment to me and treatment.

One boy, sitting on the throne he'd made, ruled as king that his separated parents would reunite. Two children tried to resolve their fear of death: one child created a live-forever box while the second went to sleep in the coffin she'd made herself. "Woof. Woof. Pat me," barked one teenager from inside her block doghouse, this play revealing the truth behind her tough, don't-need-nobody exterior. And more than one younger child has dealt with his worries about growing up by laying a block path on which he must stay lest he fall into quicksand, deep waters, and alligator-infested swamps. Children build themselves high chairs, cribs, corrals, cages, and castles. The ways our child patients use the blocks in relation to themselves are endless.

Being big, noisy (when they fall), harmless, and rather indestructible (they can support a grown man's weight), the cardboard blocks also admirably serve to express aggression.

> A shy boy, Craig gave the term *inhibited* new meaning. He spoke in almost a whisper and moved as if wrapped in a mummy suit. He seldom asked for anything and complained of little. His passivity frustrated his family, teachers, and friends beyond belief. His seemingly quiet and selfless posture somehow made more noise and called more attention to himself than were he able to speak his mind.
>
> In his therapy Craig built small and solid towers that, though they reached only to my waist, he worried might fall on and kill me. Gingerly, he would tap them, each time diving to the ground to withstand the earthshaking avalanche his projected rage caused him to anticipate. Gradually he built much higher towers that he knocked down with gusto.

Just as gradually, Craig came to talk and laugh more loudly, move more robustly, protest, and just plain feel stronger and better. The blocks provided a lively and safe forum in which to begin experimenting with the intense anger and frustration that he held so tightly inside himself. Of no surprise, the people in Craig's life found his noisy and complaining self much easier and more enjoyable to be with, a self that soon quieted not out of fear but out of genuine contentment and greater confidence.

More reckless children can exercise their self-control by toppling towers that we build or by ruining only parts of a structure, for example, or by having to describe their aggressive intent verbally before acting on it. Blocks make good targets for punching, kung fu'ing, and—a favorite of the children—pretend blowing up. Block houses can be kicked apart, huffed and puffed down by a demonic wolf, and destroyed by acts of war and Mother Nature.

Early in my practice, I discovered that the box of dominoes on my desk, rarely used to play the actual game, were constantly used to build knockdowns. Soon after, I put several more boxes of them into a straw basket that's become a staple of my playroom. Children even construct intricate designs while talking. This play is the ultimate activity for children who are prone to overwhelming frustration, for these knockdowns often fall from the slightest misstep or push on the desk.

For similar reasons, I have wooden blocks from the recycling shop of Boston's Children's Museum. My blocks are all different sizes, no two alike. Children who may find the asymmetry originally annoying soon find them interesting and a challenge that further promotes their growing easier with frustration, imbalance, and the imperfection of life. These blocks also have given children with shaky esteem an opportunity to good-naturedly belittle my toys and the therapy as secondhand and defective, making for good lead-ins to their looking at why they need to see themselves in such a critical light.[2]

GUNS

On top of old Smokey,
all covered with blood,
I shot my poor teacher,
with a 40-foot gun.
I went to her funeral,
I went to her grave,
Instead of flowers,
I brought a grenade.
But in the morning,
she wasn't quite dead,
So I took a bazooka,
and blew off her head.

Appalled? What kind of child would say, no less think, such a thing? A vicious hooligan, probably, perhaps one who's already done his share of fighting and violence. A deranged product of society? The offspring of an absent father? Maybe this child was abused. What else could account for such sick and malevolent feeling?

Actually, this was told to me by a sweet, kind, honest, hardworking young girl who wouldn't have hurt a fly if her life depended on it. She was a helpful daughter and a devoted grandchild and took reliable care of the family pets. She came to therapy because she worried too much. She worried that she and those she loved might die. She worried that everything might go wrong. And most of all, she worried that her human less-than-saintly thoughts meant she was a bad girl who deserved to be severely punished. (Incidentally, like everyone else, our young poet's teacher liked her very much and thought her a jewel in her class.)

I introduce this discussion of guns somewhat provocatively for the topic has understandably grown quite controversial over the past years. Toy guns, once every boy's right, have been banished by many. I recall reading a national ad by a major stuffed-animal manufacturer that asked, "Is it any wonder that our prisons are full?" above pictures of a green toy grenade, a blue plane, a red-and-white-striped rocket, a camouflaged army tank, and a water pistol.

If raising a healthy and decent human being only could be accomplished by purchasing the right toy! Can a small, plastic water gun truly obliterate the positive influence of a loving, respectful, and consistent upbringing? And what feeble power can a fleecy lamb wield in the face of a neglecting and abusive home? I've worked with violent children who since birth had owned stuffed animals—nice ones, too. Some of them had tortured these toys with real hammers, knives, and picks as toddlers before they'd ever laid their hands or eyes on a play weapon. Each and every one of these children came from horrible circumstances.

Whether or not we like to see or feel its presence, aggression is everywhere, throughout the world, at home, and within each of us. Our job as therapists is to help children grow into comfortably nonviolent adults who can solve their needs and problems constructively. How can children come to terms with something considered alien, nonexistent, or worthy of permanent exorcism (as if that were possible)? Both ignoring and freely expressing one's aggression represent easy ways out. Struggling to better understand and manage it is a much harder task but well worth the effort in its benefit to each of us individually and as a society.

Is it any surprise that many of the parents who've criticized my having toy guns have had children whose anger has been wholly out of control? Consider Tucker.

When Tucker's parents came to me, his public first-grade classroom was feeling unable to keep him there. A big child, he was forever bullying other children, especially those younger and smaller than he. If he felt sufficiently slighted or unattended to—which didn't take much—he'd strike out, often viciously, kicking a child even after there'd been a surrender and supposed treaty. But the main reason his parents had brought him to me was his thwarted attempt to push his baby brother's carriage off a ledge.

Although the majority of children who come to me with heady reputations prove to be rather meek and pliable in the therapy hour, Tucker
treated me no better than the others in his life. He tried to break toys,
constantly put me down, and bragged of the violent things he'd do to all
who got in his way. In his play Tucker frenetically created "Crazy Town,"
a place where everyone was vulnerable to abuse and mistreatment.

In our first month together, we began to see progress. Tucker broke
less and ranted more. He cried several times about how crazy he gets. He
even said, explicitly, that he wanted help. However, his parents, seeing
that I had toy guns in my office, became quite critical and challenging
of me. Although I empathized with their philosophy about guns in our
society, I tried my best to explain how my Nerf blaster—a long plastic
orange tube with a bright yellow push plunger—was a healthy, harmless
toy that looked nothing at all like a real gun. I could have lived without
that toy if it would have eased their minds, but Tucker's parents asked
that I not allow their son to even play out aggression in his therapy. My
best attempts to convey understanding failed, and these parents pulled
their child out of treatment.

Although there was clearly more to their agenda, Tucker's parents
expressed an increasingly common attitude toward play guns: that they
are bad, that they confuse children, that they foster violence and violent
solutions to life's problems, and that they negate goodness, caring, and
love. I can grasp that attitude unquestionably. But the truth, at least in
therapy, is different.

Play guns are first and foremost, if not exclusively, a way to express
hostility. It's that simple. I have never seen a child use a gun to talk, to
eat food with, to write with, or to make a sheltering home out of. Almost
always children use the gun to shoot; occasionally, when they miss, they
use the gun to whack down their targets. But if aggression is such a part
of the human experience and its control is so critical yet perilous, aren't
toys that advance its mastery to be applauded?

Lev had a fierce temper and was prone to letting his anger out on
whoever was handy, a playmate, a sibling, a parent, or even a teacher.
On the flip side, when he wasn't irate, he tended to be timid and
withdrawn, apt to be bullied himself. Like Tucker's mother, Lev's
mother was adamantly opposed to toy weapons. Even after Lev showed
me his anger by kicking a heating baseboard off the wall, she feared

that playing with my toy gun might make him gun-happy and more comfortable with violence. Upon seeing my toy gun, she was aghast and openly confessed her confusion. She wanted him to get my help but was upset by what she saw.

Unlike Tucker's mother, Lev's mother could see a distinction between her attitude in general and her son's therapeutic needs. She also was aware that her opinion might reflect her own issues around aggression. Over the course of her son's useful treatment, she came to see how her worldview derived from her having lived with an abusive father and her seeing men, even her beloved son, as inherently evil. While helping her to understand her son's anger as well as her own, our good work together did not erode her broader values and battle against guns, nuclear power, and war in general. In fact, in the course of growing much more comfortable with her son's play, even with toy guns, she found the truer source of her conflicts and channeled her public efforts toward supporting a shelter for women who'd been abused.

Ironically, it is often the children who exhibit intense and dangerous outbursts in their lives who are most wary of playing with my toy guns. They shoot hesitantly and quickly toss the gun down, so fearful are they that their hostile impulses will get out of hand. These children especially benefit from play with the gun, learning to shoot more vigorously without losing all control and without shooting at my face.

Just as games can loosen children's self-revelations, shooting can tap children's anger, the safeness of this expression often leading them to talk more freely about what bothers and enrages them.

Kenny presented as the most generous and caring young man. An eighth grader, he did well in school and was a good friend and son. However, he suffered intense jealousy of a younger sister that drove him to treat her miserably, often bordering on the abusive.

When asked about her, Kenny nearly always denied any feeling, claiming that she was a good sister whom he liked. It was only after weeks of his staging a shooting gallery of bear figures that he, unable to hit the little girl bear, began a tirade about his resentment over little girls. A creature of habit, Kenny spent each of his succeeding hours shooting at this little figure. As he spoke more and more openly of his envy of his sister and his fear that she was loved more, he made room for the guilt-ridden and loving feelings he'd long ago lost touch with.

Feelings of insignificance, injury, neglect, and powerlessness often fuel the abuse and violence that pervade modern life; it's no different with many of the children we treat. Thus, when children come to us ready for a good fight, we try to keep in mind the inner hurt and sense of small-ness that likely propels their need to flaunt a big gun. "Wow, you are so big and powerful," I'll first comment to a child who proudly wags the big gun between his legs, before I'll try to explore what experiences are making him feel so little. "With a weapon like that no one can hurt you," I'll note with admiration to a child who sits behind his block fortress, his gun vigilantly aimed outward.

If a play gun is to help a child manage his aggression, limits are of course critical. I don't allow shooting guns to be shot at me. I offer them large action figures as my surrogates, figures they can shoot to their heart's content. While I seldom interfere with the child–parent relationship—meaning I do not jump in to set limits that the parent cannot—I do not allow the child to shoot at his family or siblings. If he does, I take quick and certain responsibility for removing the gun from the child's hands. To allow him to break something or hurt somebody is destructive and countertherapeutic. With this structure the vast majority of children promptly learn how to use the toy gun responsibly and for their therapeutic welfare, though a Nerf gun and balls can hardly hurt anything.

In addition to just shooting, children often incorporate smaller play guns into their fantasy play. Children, I find, are most drawn to spy and police kits that allow them to be the good guys, notoriously fighting aggression with aggression, fire with fire, killing the bad guys before they kill us. Children also like to experiment with being the bad guys who must be tamed and shown the ways of proper civilization.

Needless to say, with gun play and almost any other play in the office, we must assess what is happening in the context of what we know about today's hour, current stresses, the child's broader circum-stances, personality functioning, and the social environment in which he lives. Would we spend hours staging gunfights with a child who'd actually shot and killed someone? No. But then the kind of child for whom gun play is wrong is probably a child who needs treatment much more intensive and behavioral than the kind of traditional play therapy described here.

NOTES

1. Jill Bellinson (2002) devotes an entire book to the developmental use of board games in child therapy, as do Schaefer and Reid (2001).

2. Child therapy is a low-tech operation. See Ginott's chapters (1961) on "Rationale for Toy Selection." Not much has changed in half a century.

Readers will find lots of ideas in Heidi Kaduson and Charles Schaefer's *101 Play Therapy Techniques* (1997, 2000a, 2003), a three-volume series; Kaduson and Schaefer's book on short-term play therapy (2000b); and Schaefer and Cangelosi's book on play therapy techniques (2002).

8

Drawing Out the Child: Artwork in Therapy

In their efforts to connect, communicate, and cope with us and their therapies, children use whatever means and resources they possess or can find. They play. They talk. And they draw. They draw little pictures and big ones. Sophisticated and primitive. Well done and much less well done. Whatever the nature of the drawing, it serves as one major conduit between the child and the therapist. This chapter examines the many functions and nuances that characterize children's art in therapy.

When first meeting our child patients, many of us offer them the opportunity to draw. We do so not only to collect what can be a rich harvest of data but also to help put the child at ease. Just as we adults typically find it easier to meet a stranger while smoking, holding a golf club, or pushing our child through the supermarket, many children feel more comfortable with us while holding a crayon. Drawing can help break the ice, providing a safe activity for child and therapist to begin getting to know one another.

We help to facilitate that goal by making our offers to draw inviting, meaning void of demand or expectation. Should we show too much enthusiasm for drawing, we risk chasing the child away or trapping the child who doesn't like to draw. "Would you like to draw? There are markers and paper should you wish at any time." Phrasing our invitation in these terms gives children the space to decline without feeling they have somehow failed or defied us early in the relationship.

Children who want to draw may ask what they should draw. Our suggesting that perhaps they might know what they'd like to draw is routine enough, their asking representing a bow to our authority or indecision on their part. Although whatever they draw will likely reveal much about themselves, what they first decide to draw will more generally reflect their wish to wow us with their ability. That is, children will often choose to draw not what will most communicate their psychological circumstances and suffering but the picture they can draw best. If it's a mean sunflower, we can bet we'll get sunflowers. Should sneakers with untied laces be their forte, we'll get sneakers.

When a girl asks or looks to us for guidance, we hedge. "It's not easy to decide, is it?" "What pictures are you thinking about?" "What would you like me to suggest?" Such casual remarks may open up some meaningful discussion about this child's difficulty deciding for herself and perhaps about her broader difficulties in life. We may find that she has dozens of good ideas but feels uncertain about asserting them for fear of displeasing us. Or she may tell us that her mind is blank and that this is a problem for her when teachers ask her to write stories or when friends want to play in fantasy. Once clear that the child needs our help, we may suggest several items (e.g., a child, a family, a tree, some place or thing you like). Intriguingly, it is often only after we've made suggestions that some reticent children suddenly come up with their own and better ideas about what to draw.

Whatever she chooses to draw and whenever in the therapy she draws it, the child's creations and creating will likely tell us much about herself. Before her crayon touches the paper, we begin to glean information. How does she prepare her work space? Does she grab a million sheets of paper while dumping the entire bucket of markers, tossing the top of the marker she's about to use on the floor? Or does she tease a single sheet of paper off the heap and line it up just the way she wants? One child draws with the first pencil she finds; another spends minutes trying out markers until she finds the right color with the right point. Does the child move at the speed of light or more like a turtle who plans its way?

Does she draw tentatively, her pencil etching barely visible, or does she wield the marker like a carving knife? Is her picture comfortably sparse like a Shaker home, or does it overflow with too much, the child compulsively filling in every last space? These observations begin to inform us about the girl's intellect, neurological abnormalities, self-discipline, work style, and, certainly, how she may approach tasks at school, particularly those involving drawing or, perhaps, written work.

How children manage their errors or changes of mind can further tell us something about themselves.

> Findlay angrily crumpled up his paper and threw it onto the pile that he'd accumulated for the past 15 minutes. When he wanted to draw me a picture of his new bicycle, Findlay made no less than two dozen attempts. Each time he hastily drew the front wheel. Once he saw that it wasn't perfectly round, Findlay would disgustedly cross out what he'd drawn and begin again. Only our first hour, this frustration prophesied Findlay's yearlong treatment as centering around harsh self-criticism and readiness to give up on himself quickly.

Every less-than-perfect stroke sent Findlay's esteem spiraling downward. Other children are as perfectionistic but not as narcissistically vulnerable. Over and over these children sketch, erase, sketch, erase. Although, like Findlay, they are ever disappointed with their drawing, they have the capacity not only to scrutinize their work but to fix it until it meets their high standards. Others do their correcting by coloring over their mistakes with bolder and bigger markers, proudly handing over drawings that are a mess. Still others who recognize that their drawing is not at all what they wished know that they lack the skill or interest in doing more. They lay down their marker and talk or play instead.

Perhaps the first thing we notice about a child's drawing is its skill level. Some children, of course, are more artistic than others. Although children's drawings can reveal something about their intellect (and there are scoring systems for extrapolating IQ from a child's drawing of a person), one needs to exercise caution. A child who is unmotivated, who dislikes drawing, or who is highly intelligent but motorically delayed can produce remarkably poor artwork suggestive of low intelligence. More definite assumptions about cognition and intellect are probably better found in their language and behavior or the therapeutic relationship or, better yet, from standardized psychological and educational testing.

As is true of most human endeavors, children who draw well generally like drawing more. However, this is not a firm principle to rely on. Children who draw poorly or hastily can come to recognize the communicative powers of drawing and often turn to it as a significant avenue for their therapy. When they feel we've noted their skills, even some accomplished artists are wont to pursue their artwork much in the spirit of Pictionary, drawing only as much and for how long as it takes to get their message across to us. However much of an advantage artistic talents can lend, fine or complex drawings are no more likely to carry or communicate meaning than are their simpler, more primitive counterparts.

Almost any drawn object or thing can tell us about our patients, but drawings of a child represent the mother lode. No other subject matter so vigorously pulls for children's perception of themselves. One bully's drawing of himself as bigger than a house suggested his narcissistic and counterphobic need not to see himself as the small child he was. A second, equally small child who lived in an overwhelmingly chaotic home out of his control portrayed the impotence he felt in a boy the size of a dandelion. A child with a muscle disorder drew a girl with puny arms, as did a boy who feared beating up the sister he felt so jealous of.

Just as we do for the real children who enter our office, we look at how these drawings of children are dressed. Are they wearing appropriate clothes for their age, the setting, and the weather? Do they wear clothes whose colorfulness contrasts with their own dark apparel and mood? Or is there a figure dressed in black, as if mourning? Does that boy have a tattoo that says "Mom" on his arm, and is that girl wearing a sexy evening gown to school? Do the children in the pictures appear their age, well cared for, happy? Children who are drawn nude or with invisible clothes are of particular concern, as they tend to speak to issues of reality testing, abuse, and perceptions of exquisite exposure and shame (though, of course, not necessarily).

The affect displayed, incidentally, may not seem to directly reflect what a child feels. A happy-go-lucky girl standing amid butterflies may tell us about a happy-go-lucky girl who loves nature, a sad girl who would like to be a happy-go-lucky girl who is at home with nature, or—and by no means the only alternative explanation—an abused and angry girl who, resentful that she was robbed of her happy-go-lucky butterfly of a childhood, feels too afraid or mistrustful to share it.

The portrayed child often exhibits unmistakable qualities that tell of its creator. One boy who I later learned wanted dearly to be a girl drew a boy wearing a ruffled and flowing skirt. An adorable and petite adolescent girl, feeling the onslaught of puberty, drew herself as a bloated young woman embarrassed by her burgeoning sexuality (see Drawing 8.1). A raging girl whose neglecting mother demanded her politeness drew a shark whose teeth she covered with a mask.

Needless to say, we look at the setting and context of drawings. A child about to be guillotined paints a different picture than a child on an Olympic gold medal pedestal. Seeing a child aboard a colorful Noah's Ark worries us less than seeing that child in a dilapidated lifeboat drifting alone on a stormy sea. Seeing scene in which a child takes positive, self-protective action (e.g., slays a fiery dragon) similarly encourages us more than the child who helplessly screams from the attic window of a burning house.

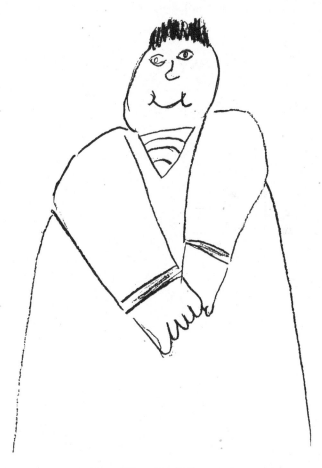

Drawing 8.1

Some children prefer to draw animals. Despite the difference of species, the self-revelations can be just as salient. One third grader, referred for poor self-esteem secondary to a learning disorder, drew a dinosaur "too stupid to add one plus one" (see Drawing 8.2). Some weeks into treatment, a depressed boy, unable or unwilling to talk with anyone, including me, drew a possum who, the child told me, wished it could just crawl back into its mother's pouch, evoking significant discussion of his understandable reaction to having been raised by a depressed and unavailable mother (see Drawing 8.3). We also see lots of cuddly bunnies, puppies, and other baby animals to represent children's longing for love and nurturance.

The atmosphere of a drawing also makes us wonder. Why is that suicidal girl drawing pictures of a sun-drenched farm? Because that's where she wants to live? Because she thinks that's what we want? Because she's not

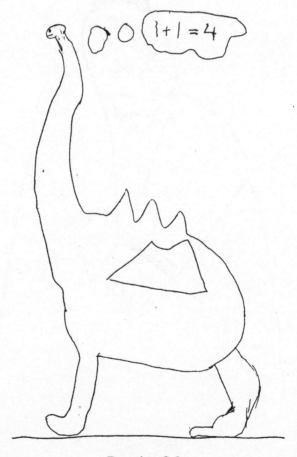

Drawing 8.2

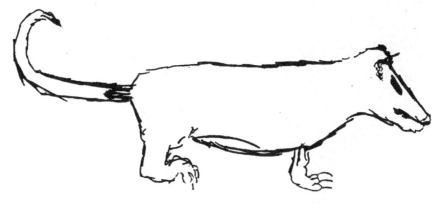

Drawing 8.3

sure she can show us what she really feels? Or, as it turned out, because she wanted to make the point of just how deceptively wonderful the relative's home where she was abused appeared to the world? Do the houses look inviting, scary, decrepit? Fire shooting from the windows means something very different from smoke curling up from the chimney.

One doesn't need to be a psychologist to know that dark skies often signal gloom and doom, as do clouds and rain often signify tears and sadness. Cold and dark often accompany loneliness, unless of course the child is portrayed snuggled cozily and happily under a blanket beside a loved parent and in front of a crackling fireplace. Is the child personified as a country or city mouse? And those natural disasters kids draw. What do they mean? Is that volcano telling us something about an overly self-controlled adolescent's mounting fury or his fear of his father's wrath, or, as happens so commonly, is it about both? I've found earthquakes, lightning, floods, and meteor collisions to be common themes in children's drawings.

> Rosalie drew a very nice picture of a very nice day. All seemed well until I asked about the hole in the tree and learned that was where "a baby squirrel was left to starve and rot" over the winter. That awful image and not the happy sunshine was what occupied this grossly neglected girl's work with me (see Drawing 8.4).

We know of course that children's drawings often tell us about life at home with the family. We take care to note whom the child's figure stands next to and whom it is isolated from. Why is the child's figure bigger than the shriveled parents (because they aren't present or able to discipline)? We can't help but be curious when one parent is drawn

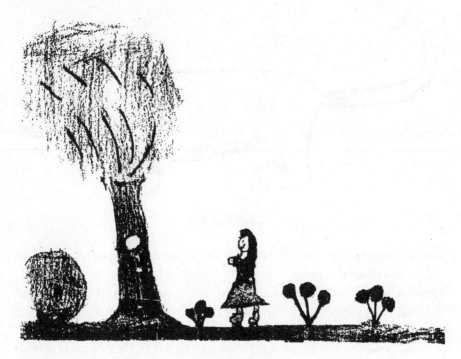

Drawing 8.4

strikingly larger than the other (more loved, more effective, or more feared and abusive?).

What is the family doing? Partaking in a fun family activity or cooperatively cooking dinner? Or does the picture depict children getting into trouble while a drinking father and crying mother fight in the kitchen? Are characters, especially the child's, distinct from others? The confusing merging of a grown child and mother can be worrisome, as can a child's continually redefining and redrawing one family member as another. Just as we observe everything about the children our child patients draw, we look carefully at their portrayals of parents and other significant people in their lives. Although a she-devil mother with horns may reflect neither a bad mother nor a disturbed son, we nonetheless tuck that little piece of data away as we proceed with the child's self-exploration.

In addition to what is in the picture, we might be equally interested in what isn't there.

In the final hour of his successful therapy, Eric drew me a picture of a helicopter hovering about the water (see Drawing 8.5). A ladder hung

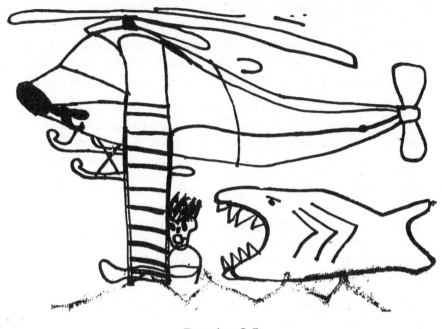

Drawing 8.5

from the helicopter, and a terrified man dangled just inches from a hungry shark's toothy mouth. It was only after most of the hour that we discovered the secret message in Eric's good-bye card to me. No one was flying the helicopter. Eric, in his poignant drawing, had shown precisely his feeling, his fear that living life without my guidance and support, without me in the cockpit, would be precarious and catastrophic. Fortunately—and to his astonishment—he did fine flying solo.

Similarly, when a child drawn in a picture seems to look askance or off to the side, I may ask, "What's the child looking at?" Intrigued by my strange question and liking the side-handed interest I'm showing, children usually come up with an answer that is worth our time. Should a gun be shooting, "Where, to what target are those bullets aimed." Babies without parents, houses without windows. I question anything that lacks what it usually has.

As with every communication, we can assume that what children draw us or in our presence has some meaning to the relationship. Snails burrowed in their shells and bears peering out from caves make me wonder whether a child is having some doubts about the spotlight of therapy and perhaps of life. When a young girl draws a young girl who asks in a speech balloon, "Am I pretty?" I must wonder if she's asking me. And can a child's vehement request that I rip up and discard a drawing of a boy covered with acne, boils, prickles, quills, and poison not say something about his self-disgust and his disbelief that I could want to do anything but dispose of him from my office and the relationship?

> Eleven-year-old Vicky had been abused for some time earlier in her childhood. Although she had every reason to be enraged and defiant, she was thoroughly compliant and made every effort to please everyone, including me as her therapist. She ceaselessly made me "I love you" cards adorned with chains of hearts and drew pictures full of happy times and happy people. Any observations I made about the compulsiveness of this artwork seemed only to make her anxious, ratcheting the level of her drivenness up a notch. Not until well into her therapy, after she'd grown sufficiently trusting, did she come to understand that she went overboard on the love cards out of fear that I would abuse and hurt her like others had.

Often times, children's drawing functions to express things that are hard to express otherwise.

> Thad, a sixth grader at a special school, could become floridly psychotic under stress. Unwanted aggressive and sexual thoughts tortured him, as did a pervasive sense of himself as massively defective and repugnant. So blinded was he by the cataclysmic flaws that he saw in himself (and that he imagined the world saw, too), he had no awareness of his formidable intellect and strengths.
>
> Prior to our working together, horrifying ideation and impulses often flooded Thad, leading to self-destructive behaviors. As his therapy evolved, however, he came to use drawing as a reliable and safe means of sharing his inner world, a world that was too complex, primitive, and, he judged, diseased to speak aloud. By using his drawings as containers and springboards for his tumultuous conflicts (e.g., his depiction of a sadistic gender-changing clinic), Thad was able to exercise greater self-control, enabling constructive work in therapy.

Sometimes what the child can't express directly may not be crazy but may be intolerably painful.

> Ryan, a first grader, was confused. He had never known his biological father, and he was glad that his mother had finally married. Moreover, he was very fond of his stepfather, a good man who was devoted to both Ryan and his mom. Because of this, Ryan did not understand the intense jealousy that he'd begun to feel since the wedding.

It was a drawing that shed light on Ryan's pain (see Drawing 8.6). That palpable caricature of Ryan's oedipal plight—his being locked out of a bedroom in which he fantasized his mother and stepfather had sex—taught us both that what had really gotten Ryan's goat was that he could no longer go in and out of his mother's room as he'd long grown accustomed to doing. This led to broader, useful discussions about the many ways Ryan now had to share his kingdom.

The unspeakable is not always ugly or taboo, either. Sometimes it's the wonderfulness, the wholesome specialness, of what the child thinks or feels that words alone can't express.

Guy, a teenage boy with Down syndrome, seldom drew. He didn't like to draw, as it came very difficult to him. But he came to one session needing to draw. He worked for most of the hour, painstakingly drawing something that I couldn't decipher.

"There's something you really want me to understand," I said.

"Yes, I do," Guy crowed, his eyes watering. With my patient query and help, he explained his drawing, a blueprint of the home he would like to have as an adult. With great pride and satisfaction, he pointed

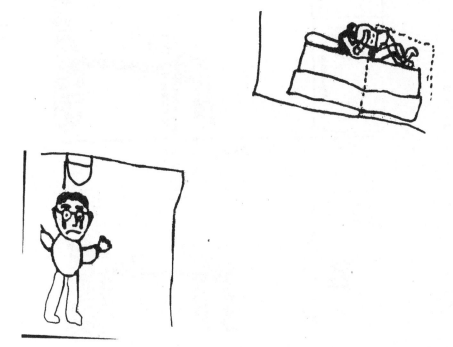

Drawing 8.6

out its quintessential feature. "See, it has wheels," he said, "so my parents can pull it behind their car." This wonderful image was Guy's fantastic and moving solution to his ambivalent wish and fear of growing up and away from his parents.

While a vast majority of children's artworks are one-shot deals meant to facilitate a moment soon to pass, a child occasionally uses a series of drawings as part of an ongoing leitmotif to his therapy.

Leroy, a high-functioning autistic boy, dealt with his transfer from another therapist to me by creating detailed schematics of the old sub-way line that brought him to therapy and the new line that was replac-ing it. Each week, for months, Leroy would build one more station

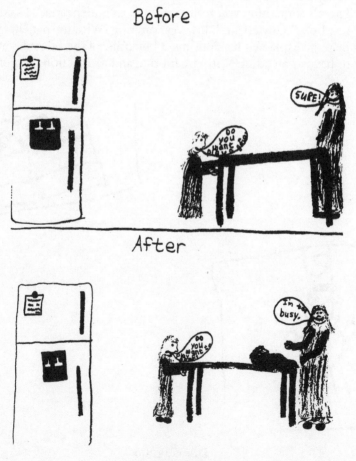

Drawing 8.7

that, over many months, was assembled into a subway world that integrated the two lines, the old and the new, allowing for his fantasy of being able to use the new line (and new therapist) without having to wholly give up the old line (and therapist before me). (Bromfield, 2007, Chapter 5)

The creative and unpredictable ways in which children use drawings to further their therapies is impressive. One girl whose sibling envy had reached meteoric proportion drew before-and-after pictures that showed, more vividly than 10,000 words could have, how her life had come undone by her sister's birth (see Drawings 8.7 and 8.8). No less dramatically did her clever use of a no-babies-allowed-here symbol illustrate her

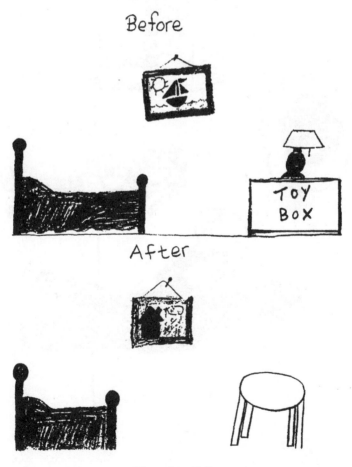

Drawing 8.8

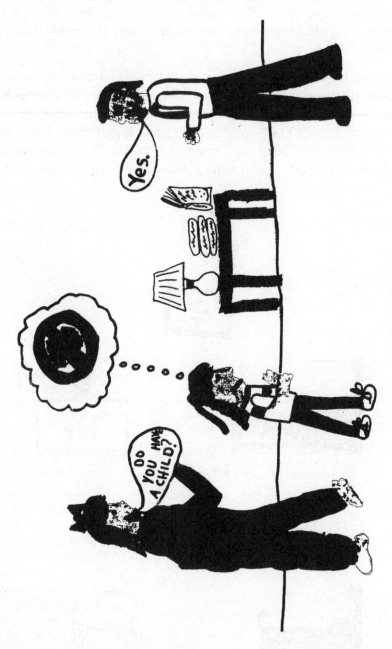

Drawing 8.9

wish that her sister had never been born (see Drawing 8.9). Wanting to convince me of just how nasty and perilous life could be at his home, one boy drew me hazardous mazes from which I could not escape death and other mishap (see Drawing 8.10).

Could words have expressed the preoccupied neglect that one artistic teenager felt as embodied in his spontaneous drawing of his "family's mind-set" (see Drawing 8.11)? Another youngster, wanting to show me more of his hidden thoughts, drew a boy and an X-ray close-up of what

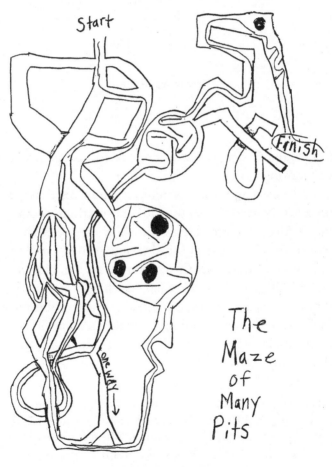

Drawing 8.10

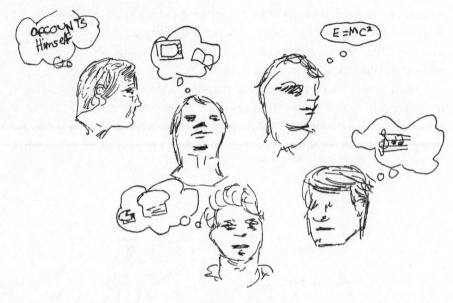

Drawing 8.11

he carried around in his pocket (a prelude to his opening up in treatment; see Drawing 8.12).

That how we treat and react to children's drawings makes a difference will surprise no clinician. Open to reading everything and anything into what children draw, we are careful with how we use what we find. We do not report sexual abuse over one drawing of an evil-looking man (for, incidentally, we may learn that the child portrays us). Nor do we barrage a drawing with 20 questions. We keep hunches to ourselves, probing or interpreting our suspicions with caution and when an abundance of clues accumulate. Overzealous trampling on children's drawings is the surest way to kill its displacing function, making drawing one more place where the child feels unsafe.

Seven-year-old Terrence showed me a picture of a child trying to win a ski race (see Drawing 8.13). "The winner gets his mother to give him a special snack," he explained. Although the mountain did appear to be somewhat of a breast, I refrained from saying so. When

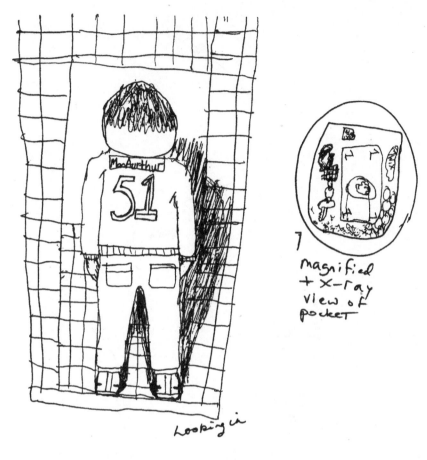

Drawing 8.12

he asked me if I'd like to see a close-up of the "most wonderful mountain in the world," however, I said that I would, only to find clear confirmation of my speculation (see Drawing 8.14). These telling drawings catalyzed Terrence's more direct discussion of the longing for nurturance from a mother who was narcissistically unavailable.

However fun and appealing, drawing is no more or less another realm in which the child can express herself within the therapy. As with any

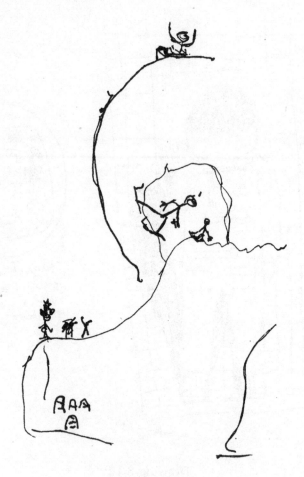

Drawing 8.13

other precious thing the child says or plays out, what she draws is subject to our careful observation and gentle pursuit. Whatever the subject or manner of her drawing, we treat it as a communiqué, one whose meaning we work to understand. As part and parcel of our relationship and the therapy, children's artwork is fair game for all of the vigilant watching, thinking about, and intervening that we as child therapists employ in our endeavor to help children know themselves better and more comfortably.[1]

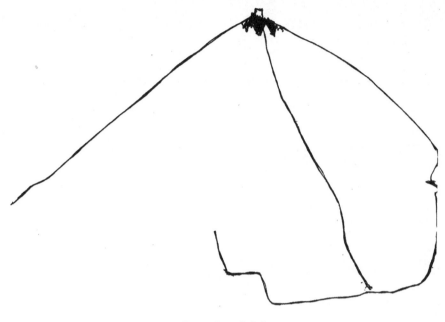

Drawing 8.14

NOTE

1. The children who come to see us regularly draw and use art to express themselves, and yet child therapists tend to get little formal training in this area. We can learn much from the field of art therapy. Good sources include Klorer (2000), Malchiodi (1997, 1998), Riley (1999), Rubin (2005), and Schroder (2004). Readers might wish to check out the web page and resources of the American Art Therapy Association (www.artherapy.org). Readers might also find interest in the case study and drawings of an artistic girl who communicated near exclusively through her art (Bromfield, 2006).

9

All Together Now: Balancing Play and Talk

Children in therapy play. They also talk. While each in itself communicates and does the work of therapy, it is the interplay between them that endows play therapy with its richness and power. As therapists, how we deal with this sometimes vigorous, sometimes delicate balance is essential. How do children and therapists use the world of play and talk to its fullest?

Children vary in their capacities to talk and play. Some can play the dickens out of life and therapy. But they will avoid more direct discussion of themselves as if it were the plague. Other children talk easily but can't play. Some do both with ease and pleasure; some do neither. What do these tendencies tell us and what should we do about them, if anything?

Seldom is a child's wish and ability to play a bad thing. Being a second and effective avenue for self-expression and communication, the gift of play generally makes therapy easier and more appealing. Our play materials announce to the playful girl that this is her kind of place and makes for a good beginning toward her ultimate ownership of the office and therapy. We all know such children, and most of us feel encouraged when we meet them. These are the children who run to our toy boxes or spontaneously grab a dog puppet to bark at us when we've asked the first question they prefer not answering. Whatever the substance of therapy and its parallel relation to the matter of life, these children seem to get it even before we demonstrate it. "We're here to be with you," they appear to know, "and we can use whatever we want, however we want, to aid that endeavor."

Not every child, however, sees toys as delicious. Some perceive our playthings to be discomforting demands. The very playthings we hope will engage them make some children feel they are in just one more place that will make them feel inadequate for not playing like a child should. That children who can't play are often uncomfortable interacting with people only accentuates their feeling out of place. And while making clear that children who don't want to or can't play are equally welcome here—staying put in our chairs, not trying to sell our toys too enthusiastically—can provide some needed and early relief, it begs the question as to the larger therapy.

> First-grader Jeff showed no interest in my toys. In his second hour he'd carefully surveyed them, but over the next several months didn't look at them again. There he sat for weeks of sessions, in the overstuffed chair across from my own, looking like a miniature adult—upright, rather still, and willing to discuss the reasons his mother had brought him to me.
>
> A most serious and articulate only child, it was easy to see that Jeff carried the weight of the world on his smaller-than-average shoulders. His intellectual precocity and watchful nature and his being parentified by an overwhelmed single mother made for a child who knew too much, who was prematurely disillusioned, and who'd, to some degree, been losing out on the more innocent and free-living parts of childhood. Initially, when listening to Jeff talk about his difficulties, I wanted to throw him gleefully into the toy box. "Play! Play, little boy." But I knew that would have traumatized him; at least for the time being, he could not play.
>
> Like two adults, we sat and talked of his worries about himself as well as his greater and justified worries concerning his mother. We talked about his contempt for children who do nothing but watch

television, play video games, and draw "stupid" pictures. He "had more important things to do," though he could never say what they were. Worrying, I suspect, was one of them. Our talking helped Jeff grow less worried, less tense, and considerably happier as well as more interested in playing on his own and with other children outside of therapy.

But Jeff didn't lay a hand on my toys until the last session of a planned termination. "You've got some pretty cool stuff," he noted as he rummaged through my toys. "It's too bad I never played with them."

"And with me?" I asked, my remark causing Jeff to cry and nod his head.

"I wish my mom would have liked playing with me."

Jeff used his therapy essentially to talk through his not being able to play and his being raised by a mother whose own stresses and depression deprived him of the natural joy and responsiveness that makes for a good childhood. Each week's insights enabled him to play more freely outside the office and allowed him to take and enjoy the attentiveness that people other than his mother might offer. By not playing with me, by not indulging that longing, he constructively and unusually kept his therapeutic nose to the grindstone, analyzing, if you will, his frustrating plight right up to the final moment.

Conversely, there are children whose talent for fantasy, charming and intriguing as it is, somehow brings less insight and progress than the wonder and passion of their play might suggest.

"Satan boy" was a dramatic story that 10-year-old Gregory played for months. Each week the plot thickened, seeming to grow tighter and more to the emotional points that fueled it. Yet as far as we could see, there were no therapeutic benefits accompanying this play. Gregory left sessions appearing no lighter than when he came. School and the home front were status quo with bad news.

My attempts to move the play, enter it, or look at it were rebuffed. Like an eccentric cousin who won't let anyone get a word in edgewise, Gregory played at full speed, going around and under me as he needed, my presence more like an obstacle to the personal theater he staged. It was paradoxically only when—his parents about to halt the treatment— that I halted his play as a last-ditch effort. His therapy took off.

"You can't do this," the ever pleasant Gregory yelled. "I can do whatever I want. It's my hour."

I stood my ground.

"It's my time. I don't care what you say. I'm playing anyway." Although Gregory protested loudly, he made no move toward the toys or "Satan boy." By the hour's end, Gregory, having lambasted me with a sharp tongue worthy of "Satan boy" himself, was in tears. "You're no better than my parents. You don't care what I want. You only care about yourself."

When Gregory returned the following week, he went right to work on "Satan boy," and I did nothing to stop him. We'd made an important transition together, and he, though playing out the same fantasy, no longer had to lock me out. Having stated directly his smoldering sentiment, he no longer had to dedicate his play to passively denying me my watch and query and denying himself the comfort and help of therapy.

The example of Gregory is one reason why I feel the humanistic child-centered view, though dear to the evolution and practice of child therapy, is in itself not quite enough. Establishing a safe atmosphere in which Gregory could be himself allowed him to play in his self-absorbed and controlling way, a way he would have continued forever, or at least for many more months, by which time his parents would have stopped bringing him. Providing an accepting environment in which he could blossom hadn't sufficed; exposing himself and his hurts was just too much. My standing in the way of his playing and interrupting his natural pace, steps that run contrary to the tenets of humanistic child therapy, were what pushed Gregory and his therapy onward.

Comparably, we often meet children whose play moves so fast and wildly that we are at a loss to know what it means and what we should do. These children, who can fantasize with the prolificacy and terror of Stephen King's fiction, play, play, and play!

The play of Peter, an impulse-ridden and occasionally psychotic third-grade boy, resembled an epic nightmare staged by 1930s Hollywood. For instance, in one hour "Cookie Man" stole all the cookies of the world (Peter was neglected and needy) mostly to deprive one little girl (he was also very jealous of his newborn sister) who was kidnapped by cannibals (oral aggression—biting, spitting, and cursing were problem behaviors) but didn't die because in the meantime Peter's attention turned to a village of stupid, happy people (Peter disdained peers he saw to be happy or earnest) that was being studied secretly by a mad scientist who appeared to be a caring man but really had evil intentions (me, his object of fear in addition to himself) and who was making a super nuclear bomb (Peter was acutely aware and frightened about America's situation with Iraq as well as his own colossal hostility) that went up into space until. . . .

This play occurred in a 10-minute span, if that. By the time Peter's right hand had set up some scene, his left was replacing it with another, this pace continuing, even accelerating, as the hour raced to its end. Every conflict he played out engendered others, all of which screeched for expression like hungry chicks. So intense was the push of his internal world that the limitations of the external one mattered little. If Peter suddenly thought of death and needed a coffin, he'd grab the nearest object. Unlike the child who wants every plaything to be in realistic proportion, Peter preferred to use a pencil as a coffin (to awkwardly lay a dead figure on) than to spend a moment searching for a box or making one. More acutely, it was less a matter of preference and more one of irrepressible need.

At first I tried to enter his play world, but that failed. By the time I got there, which was fairly quickly, his play was somewhere else, causing me to literally and psychically miss the boat. Remarking on the specifics of his play—"Cookie Man sure is hungry," "Cookie Man wants all the cookies for himself"—went nowhere, for in the moments it took me to conceive and speak my thoughts, his mind and issues had moved on. In a psychic form of the Heisenberg principle, Peter's play, his electron of fantasy, could not be fixed in time and space. And if my missing the mark wasn't bad enough, my fumbling intrusions only stressed him, giving him more feelings to deal with in his play.

Much of what he did was incoherent. His play baffled me. There were far too many characters to analyze, and each one, I knew, was a most complicated mixture of people and projections. And so, unable to intervene on the specifics of Peter's play, I instead remarked on its process.

"Wow! So much happens and so quickly."
Peter sighed. "It's not easy playing like this."

For months I sat back, saying but a few words each hour, mostly at the end, words meant to capture the spirit of the whole hour. "My gosh. Murder, cancer, kidnapping, babies born, babies dying, schools exploding."

"Peter, it's astonishing. At 4:00 we started in Boston, and by 4:50 we'd traveled to every continent, outer space, and inside a volcano." Peter listened intently to what I said. Gradually his play slowed, grew more cohesive, employed fewer and fewer figures, and allowed me to join in. After the first session in which he invited me to play, Peter acknowledged that however hard playing like this was, living like this was even harder.

The zest and whimsy of play and our adult-centric overvaluing of talk can sometimes lead us to forget that what children play can be as serious as what they speak, if not more so.

Barry was an exceedingly bright 11-year-old who suffered pervasive anxiety and incapacitating phobias involving germs and illness. For weeks he talked in a pseudomature and emotionless way about his fears. That discussion brought him no apparent relief. In the final minutes of his fifteenth hour, however, he nonchalantly made a toy woman drink from my tiny teacup. The woman died. "Your cup was probably poisoned," he explained.

Barry seemed to speak about everything, everything except his greatest immediate fear that my toys were germ-ridden and that playing with them would make him sick and possibly kill him. But only through his small play gesture could he express that morbid worry and open the door to a resolution of his even bigger troubling thoughts and anxieties. For Barry, talk usually equaled an intellectual activity devoid of feeling. It was his play that ultimately allowed his worried fantasies to surface and be mastered.

Whereas the allure of rich fantasy play can make us forget the therapeutic need for discussion, play that is tedious and repetitive can lead us to overly push the child to talk.

"You be the truck and I'll be the car." Trevor had played this game for seven straight hours, each hour seeming to be a carbon copy of the last. "I'll crash into you and you crash into me." And so, for yet another hour, we did the same.

We might as well have been clicking ballpoint pens for 50 minutes once a week, it seemed to me. I found myself dreading Trevor's hour. Clinically speaking, I couldn't see what I was doing to help him behaviorally or to advance his self-exploration.

In his eighth hour, after just a minute or two of his same old my-car-crash-your-car play, I pushed the cars aside. "What's bugging you?" I asked, thinking that my straight talk would glide through his guard, bringing his conflict to the forefront for our dismantling. But it didn't. Trevor began to cry, but not the kind of cry that is relieving or connecting. My assault on him had frightened him. Being with me in therapy was stressful enough. I'd pushed him over the edge. He spent the remainder of the hour withdrawn in a far corner of the office, unwilling to talk or to play.

"What had happened?" I found myself wondering as his next hour approached. I realized that my too-to-the-point query and decision that he and I must talk was not as much clinically guided as it reflected my hostility. "What's bugging *me*?" was the question that needed asking. I began to acknowledge how enormously irritated I felt when with him, particularly when he crashed his car into mine, feeling like someone who'd been getting head-slapped over and over again. Much more than boring me, he'd been passively shutting me out of his life and it bothered me.

In his ninth hour I had the cars laid invitingly on the desk before his return. Armed with my self-understanding, Trevor's crash play no longer seemed to annoy me. It was no longer a personal thing. I recognized that he had to fend me off: closeness was the feared enemy. Reading accurately that he could play crashing as long as he wished and that it no longer bugged me, Trevor soon went onto more freed up play and talk.

The meaning of a child's playing or not playing, talking or not talking, is steeped in the finite context of the moment as well as in the child's bigger situation, in who the child is psychologically and the relativity of what the child is doing or not doing now compared with what she usually does and what she did last. Two spoken lines may be nothing more than a couple of grace notes for the child who talks nonstop through the therapy hours. For a second child, who tends only to play, those few words can speak a symphony.

A child's playing or talking can take on special meaning when its characteristic pattern changes. While playing board games can be a disheartening sign that one child continues to stall self-analysis, it can herald the good news that a second borderline and fantasy-fraught child's ego has grown sufficiently to allow him to sit peacefully and play a game. Similarly, while a tumultuous earthquake striking the dollhouse may just be one more instance of a violent child's play, it can be an indication that a neurotically inhibited child is getting better.

Short time-frame transitions between talk and play can carry special meanings.

> Stuart had worked hard for more than half an hour setting up a massive army of soldiers, townspeople, and policemen to battle my three large dinosaurs. Satisfied with the cast, he proceeded to play out a vicious battle that seesawed between the two forces. After five minutes, only the T-Rex and head general remained standing. Stuart raised the little soldier's right arm and sword and charged. But just before he could pierce the T-Rex, he abruptly put the toys down. "I'd better clean up," he said.
>
> "You've got almost fifteen minutes left," I said.
>
> "That's okay," he replied, his quick cleaning up telling me that he had some good reason for stopping.

Much in the way that conflicts disrupt analytic patients' free associations and motivation to do analysis, conflicts can disrupt a child's play and his motivation to do therapy. Only in the next hour did I learn what had halted Stuart. Reenacting the previous week's play, this time he focused on the duel between T-Rex and the general.

> "I didn't mean to kill you," the general cried, standing above the huge dinosaur that now lay on its side, dying with a sword through its head. "If you hadn't stolen my queen, none of this would have happened," the heartbroken general explained. "We could have been friends."

Although he liked his stepfather, Stuart didn't like the man's marrying his mother. Stuart's liking for him made him feel like a traitor to his birth father, a man who was far less adept at and invested in being a dad. Stuart couldn't play out such complex and heavy conflict easily and at once any more than an adult could tell it all during one therapy hour.

The reverse, of course, is something that happens all the time in child therapy. Ask a boy whether he's still getting detentions, and he suddenly has a burning desire to play dominoes. Sometimes the child is subtle, sometimes not. "Can't we just play?" "Do we have to talk?" Those less bound to civilities and decorum just walk away from us and our questions, playing as if we are nothing more than flies buzzing about their head. Some children—those who may be less amenable to treatment—cut us off cleanly. They go off and play without us. Others, however much they try, can't help themselves. Their play continues to deal with what it defends against or what they're trying to run from.

> Clark was in trouble. His private school was about to expel him. His after-school program already had done so. His defiance had alienated almost everyone in his life. Yet he refused to discuss any aspect of his situation, particularly his recent tendency to destroy whatever environment he was in. "I don't care," he muttered as he walked over to the toy box.
>
> But every dimension of Clark's play seemed to state that he cared very much. First, he made a big mess of the toys, dumping things everywhere in his attempt to find what he was looking for. Second, using play figures he staged a scene of a child who refused to use the toilet, pooping and peeing in the sink, in his parents' bed, and even on the Thanksgiving dinner. Third, at the hour's end the action figures voted not to clean up after themselves. Fourth, though I did not require it, he did clean up.

Clark's play essentially expressed with considerable complexity what he felt unable to put into words. Feeling empowered by my allowing him to defy my demand to talk, he began to show in his play the oppositional motive underlying his behavior. My allowing him to safely defile my office on many levels, to symbolically poop and pee on my floor and myself, he was able to look at what he'd done and to decide spontaneously to clean up after himself. Through play like this, he eventually grew to understand and master the fears evoked by his wish to be a good boy.

For many children, the displacing function of therapy—its allowing for more psychologically distanced expression of thoughts, feelings, and experiences—is well appreciated, if unconsciously, and naturally taken advantage of. But is displacement enough?

For some, like Austin, it is. Austin was referred to me after he'd been knocked off his bicycle by a neighborhood dog. The resulting phobia had increasingly closed his life in. He was afraid to leave his house, and that fear in turn induced a school phobia and a reluctance to play with friends outside of his own home.

> With the exception of my initial evaluation, and only when I asked, Austin played and talked for four months without once bringing up

dogs, dog bites, or his phobia. His play, however, overflowed with rage against his extremely controlling and angry mother. Relieving and coming to understand his own rage, the projection of which had made dogs look ominous indeed, quickly and surely undid his phobias. He left his therapy confident, his previous love of dogs wholly renewed.

Other children can play seemingly until the end of time without gaining insight, without making change, and without getting better.

Although only 11, Jared was abusive to his passive and depressed mother. Previous therapies, including family systems work and medication for his own depression, hadn't helped. Encouraged by his rich play and openness to fantasy, I eagerly worked with him for several months. Soon enough, I had to see that his playing out of abuse and strife was not helping. In fact, even after sessions in which he'd played out his mean-spirited behavior along with seemingly genuine remorse, he'd abuse his mother as they left my office.

Jared taught me that play alone, while important, is no cure-all. My work was no more helpful than the failed family work, for the same reason. Jared's parents were unable to stop their passive but sadistic treatment of each other and their torturous use of Jared as an object over which to wage their destructive and hateful war. Playing with me was merely sticking a pinky finger in a dam that burst with holes the size of basketballs. Sometimes a child's outer reality is so toxic that the child's playing it out can distract us from the harsher and bigger steps that must be taken or reckoned with.

Implicit in these discussions of talk and play is the question of whether to directly enter the child's fantasy world or to keep back and observe it. Although no guarantee that it's the right choice, children often tell us what they want.

"Just watch. I'll let you know when I need you." Sitting on the floor, Erica kept her barnyard scene sheltered within her spread legs, her body shielding what she did. My slightest movement caused her to stop playing and protectively circle her arms around her things.

Erica's behavior was not difficult to understand. Her mother was a destructively intrusive woman who, though quite sexually provocative, had never abused her. This mother routinely went through Erica's room and backpack in search of clues of drugs or sexual activity, believing she did it for her daughter's well-being. Erica welcomed the attention and help of therapy, but she feared that I would be as self-centered and manipulative as her mother. My allowing her to play safely and privately in my presence showed her firsthand that her complicated needs would be respected and met.

As much as Erica didn't want me intruding, Abby did.

"Why aren't you playing?" Abby asked me with annoyance for the fifth time in this hour.

"I'm really frustrating you."

"Yes, you are. And I'm getting tired of it."

I chose to stop trying to explain to Abby the many reasons why I hadn't been playing. Because: she'd crawled under the chair, taking all of her toys with her; grabbed an action figure from me and told me to just shut up; switched the play so abruptly that I hadn't figured out what was happening in the split second it took her to complain that I wasn't there; she'd taken her play out to the waiting room, instructing me to wait in the office. Early in our meetings I learned that telling her why I wasn't playing only made her feel blamed, frustrating her even more. She wasn't interested in what she'd contributed to my not playing; she knew only that she didn't like it.

She had good reason not to like it. Her big-time banker father seldom spent time with Abby, nor did her equally big-time executive mother. Early on, both confessed to me their "never being the kind of parents who play with their children." "Sometimes I'll read company reports while she plays next me," was how her father described their closer moments. "Children bore me," Abby's mother admitted. "It sounds awful, but that's just how I am." Was Abby responsible for her parents not playing with her, as she was with me? Not at all. What she constructively re-created with me were situations in which I was unavailable to her, and that abandonment was what she needed confirmed, understood, and help to cope with.

As therapists, especially with borderline and psychotic children—those for whom the boundaries between inner and outer reality are ill defined—we often strive to put one foot in the reality of play while keeping the second firmly on the floor of external reality.

Nick was a severely troubled eight-year-old. Under the slightest stress he was prone to lose control of himself: throwing tantrums, destroying property, aggressing against others and himself, and urinating and defecating in his pants. Of even more concern was the degree to which he suffered from poor judgment, night terrors, and unremitting self-hatred that constantly put him in peril or invited mistreatment.

The cannibals—people action figures—surrounded the little boy who was being turned on a spit above the fire. "Help me! Don't let them eat me!" Nick screamed, sounding almost as frightened as any roasting child might feel. But things on this island were not as simple as we might have wished. "He deserves to be eaten. He deserves to be sliced like bacon and fed to the meanest pigs. But," he added, "even they will probably throw him up. That's how disgusting he is."

"But I don't deserve to die," I protested for the boy figure.

"You deserve worse," Nick replied firmly.

"But no child deserves to die," I said, hoping to side with whatever tidbit of self-loving protectiveness there was in Nick.

"No child but this one." Nick would have none of my sympathy for that child.

Nick made clear that I was not to save the boy or intervene in any other way. "What do I do?" I asked, meaning it.

"You watch and suffer like everyone else." And that's just what I did. Nick reportedly had a better week after this session.

Had I suggested directly that Nick was that child being cooked, he would have disagreed vehemently and felt stripped naked by my flippant exposé. A more tactful and psychologically cautious statement—"I wonder if you sometimes feel bad enough to be cooked and eaten"—would have injured him less but felt nearly as threatening. And besides, even if my remarks could be heard, weren't they awfully narrow?

After all, was Nick merely that boy? No. He was also partly the cannibals being punished for a voracious hunger for attention, admiration, love, and all of the other human food he had long been deprived of. He was also the chief cannibal who initially judged this boy as warranting that harsh consequence. This complicated mess was yet more complicated, for Nick's wish to wholly devour (and thus possess) those he loved and depended upon—while being punished—was also being gratified, for he, as the cannibals, got to enjoy the meal.

The overarching context between the two of us carried even more meanings. I was forced to helplessly watch the scene, confused and pained. Nick particularly appreciated my being witness to this multiply leveled, polyrepresentational drama, a concrete production of the psychic horror he bore by himself almost every moment of his life. Instead of making numerous pointed comments that connected bits and pieces of his play to himself, I interpreted in a larger way what I'd seen within the play itself.

"The poor boy. The poor cannibals. The poor pigs. Everyone is miserable and no one knows why any of this misery has to happen."

Nick understood what I said instantly and with satisfaction. Without stealing the cover of play from him, without prematurely confronting him, and without neglecting the most basic truth that the story was all about him, its sole writer, actor, and director, I conveyed that I grasped what he wanted most of all: my knowing just how bloody tortured it was to be Nick.

Using what I consciously knew about Nick, I made a superficially modest statement whose underbelly spoke to all of his various levels of conflict and hurt. By talking about the play creatures as I did, taking their plight and pain as seriously as I might that of human people, I helped anchor Nick in the outer world while helping to keep him safe and sound in his just-as-real inner world. It is playing in that transitional space, the realm of play and fantasy, that enables our child patients to learn to master and reconcile what they think, feel, and imagine on the inside with the stresses, truths, and limitations of the outer world they must live in and comply with.

The relationship between talk and play also can involve the relationship between affect and thinking. All cognition and logical thinking won't do it, nor will waterfalling emotions that can neither be regulated nor processed. Children's play in treatment often, though not always, involves more energy and spontaneity than their talk does. How and why do we work to help the child connect the two?

Amy was a polite and cooperative child. She talked at length about her frustration at school and her wish not to go anymore. "I just don't feel right there," she explained calmly. "I don't know why." She spoke well only of the younger sister, whom she regularly tormented. That tormenting plus the school phobia were the reasons her parents were seeking treatment for her. Any question I asked she answered, though her responses tended to be stilted and shallow.

Amy's play was a wholly different species. Her murderous envy of her sister and the classmates with whom she had to share her teacher's attention came out loud, clear, and in brilliant technicolor. "I hate you. I hate you. I wish you were never born," she screamed at these competitors for the love she wanted to possess exclusively, her face beet red.

"No wonder school is so terrible," I said quietly.

Amy nodded agreement, heartfelt tears cascading down her cheeks.

Many of the gains Amy made in treatment came from her reuniting her emotional turmoil with her more rational thinking. That allowed her to gain understanding that provided relief and enabled her to make changes in her behavior, behavior that unbeknownst to her had been pushing away those she wanted close by. Before treatment, her formidable brain power had enabled her to adapt by relating intellectually to the world, her emotions coming forward mostly when she was overwhelmed, when she could no longer keep them to herself. As therapy proceeded, Amy's talk became more expressive and revealing, as did her thinking; her play grew less titanic. She came to live more comfortably between her inner and outer worlds as a better integrated child who could flexibly both think and feel.

Arguably the most facilitating of all the intricacies between play and talk in therapy is the creation of a shared world that serves to hold, connect with, and invite children to face their lives and themselves.

For months Maurice had built himself an entire world within the office. After experimenting with various arrangements, he'd settled on the desk as home base, the big chair becoming that of the enemy. The alcove was a magical escape hatch that offered unlimited supplies, all the information of the world, and perfect protection. When Maurice dared to leave our fort to see the world, he could enjoy all of those prizes by simply keeping even just a toe somewhere in the vicinity of that alcove. "Even atom bombs can't reach us here," he said. Within this general scene an abundance of complicated and evolving activity took place, which became increasingly organized and lasting. Each week took off where he'd previously ended.

Maurice used this ongoing play to cope with a life that was predictable only in its unpredictability. His parents were unreliable, however much they cared for him—indulgent this moment, neglectful the next. Both parents had explosive tempers and waged horrific battles in front of Maurice. The elaborate universe he created with me allowed his therapy to move smoothly and efficiently, with no waste of time, enhancing its therapeutic coherence and efficiency.

Through such enduring play or talk, children do their therapeutic work speedily and exuberantly. In fact, it can be a good sign when an obsessive boy decides that he neither wants nor needs to spend the first half of each hour recapping the one before or explaining to me every detail of what had gone before. "You remember," some children comment with surprise, happy that I care enough to listen and freed up to play more for themselves and less for me.

The pace and flow of a child's play and talk is as vital, varying, and interwoven as are the bubbling creek and the land through which it runs and percolates. It is our ongoing attention to talk and play, as well as the way they slow and ease one another, that allows us to most keenly help children to engage in their own therapy.[1]

NOTE

1. Some of the play dynamics of this chapter are found with children who have various forms of borderline organization. Despite their being somewhat dated, readers will much appreciate the insights, practicality, and timeliness of Ekstein and Wallerstein (1956), Masterson (1972), and Pine (1974) as they apply to such play and children. I give a special shout-out to Ekstein (1966), a book that, to my mind, contains all of the secrets to being an effective child therapist.

10

Pushing the Envelope: On Giving, Telling, and Other Exceptions

If we've learned anything from our work as therapists, it's how critical consistency and constancy are. Our talents for playing, communicating, and understanding play second fiddle to our ability and willingness to establish and preserve the framework of a therapy. Still, whether or not in their own best interests, our patients yell for more, for things that run against or jump over these boundaries we've worked so hard to erect and maintain. Being no less human than the children we see, we know our own wishes to get around those walls—and not only in response to our patients' requests. What do these cries, theirs and ours, for exceptions to the rule mean, and what do we do with them?

The giving of things is probably the clearest place to begin our discussion. Early in my training I routinely gave my child patients gifts on their birthdays and during the holiday season. I did it mostly because my experienced patients would cannily tell me, the beginner, about the wonderful gifts their previous therapists had given them. "Give us something good, and we'll like you as much," they seemed to say. "Or even more." My wish to make these unhappy children happy and the commonplace truth that grown-ups do buy children gifts helped to rationalize my relatively unexamined decision. Admittedly, the fact that I had only three child patients in that first practicum minimized the cost and inconvenience of buying presents. A caseload of 20 might have forced me to think through the clinical significance of my actions earlier.

My gift giving never seemed to accomplish what I'd intended. One child said a simple "Thanks" and then left the gift in my office. Another child spent his hour profusely thanking me for a gift that I could see disappointed him and left more miserable than when he'd entered. My gift was a triple burden to him: not only had I given him something he didn't like, but because he liked me and appreciated my gesture, he had to keep his upset to himself; also, my beginning his birthday hour by giving him something took the wind out of his therapeutic sails. How could he dump his sadness and anger over his family's neglect of his birthday and him on someone nice enough to bring him a present?

What does it mean to a child to be given a gift by the therapist? It can mean the obvious and generally what we wish to convey, that the therapist likes or even loves me enough to remember me in this way. This is perhaps something we want the child to feel as a so-called corrective experience. Clinically, this can most apply to the truly neglected child who also is unlikely to benefit from analyzing the lack of a therapist's gift.

Our presents can also send messages we don't intend. You've given me a gift, children can imagine, to make up for the fact that you don't know what you're doing with me; to bribe me or as a payoff for your failing me in other ways; because you give gifts to everyone and so have to give me one, too; so you won't have to deal with my aggression; so you won't have to feel my sadness; because I nagged you for one; because you pity me...

As with everything else we do and say to them, children who misread why we've given them gifts can reveal more about themselves and their experiences than about ourselves. Those who feel the ways I've just described likely have good reasons to. Children who feel we give gifts to assuage their anger may have parents who do that, or perhaps that is their own modus operandi, the reason they give gifts. Projecting their own motives onto others, manipulative children can only assume we give presents not out of pure generosity but to get something (or not get something) for ourselves or to control someone. Children who have been reared to feel guilt for whatever they receive will be prone to feel in our giving the same underlying resentment they feel in their parents'.

Although they often misperceive our giving, children can sometimes detect the unconscious reasons for our giving. While we may think we're trying to brighten a poor child's Christmas, we may be trying more to alleviate our own guilt over having much more. Are clinicians who regularly give gifts to patients exceptionally caring, or are they unknowingly ensuring, by paying this tribute, that their patients like them or be happy? What does it mean when we find ourselves pulled to give gifts to certain children and not others? The more we can tease out the reasons for our gift giving, the less likely we will divert the therapy and the more likely we will allow for and recognize the impact of our giving on the child.

Whatever our underlying motivations, receiving gifts is apt to make children feel thought of, appreciated, appreciative, and to some extent indebted. "Are these feelings that will enhance the treatment?" we ask ourselves. A child who is respected, attended to, and cared for therapeutically might already feel all the goodness that our gift intends to bring. Will a gift add to them? Or will it detract? Being given a gift can discourage some children from sharing negative thoughts about us and the therapy, not just during the birthday session but for weeks to come. "If I can keep my bad feelings to myself," they may further decide, "my therapist will be more likely to buy me something else come the next occasion." And what does this gift mean for future months and years of treatment? Giving a gift today can sometimes force a therapist into gift giving tomorrow; gift giving that feels right today may feel wholly out of clinical line in a therapeutic context that we and our patients have yet to experience.

For all of our thoughtfulness, our gift giving and refraining can lead to unexpected results.

> "I don't want it." Six-year-old Colleen panted with upset, trying to push the teddy bear back into its box as quickly as she could. "Get it away from me. I hate it."
>
> "You don't want the baby, either?" I asked, holding a smaller, identical bear. Colleen's anguished screaming answered my question. "Get them out of here!"

Adopted after a yearlong and traumatic orphaning in Asia, Colleen experienced life as if skinless. To Colleen, daily living was an endless ordeal of stress and injury. Whether coming from outside or inside, almost every feeling threatened her self and typically led to disorganizing pain and reflexive aggressing against others, property, or herself. Having made considerable progress on her capacity to attach with her most dependable mother and very connected with me and therapy, I'd hoped that the mother–baby bear would be a perfect Christmas gift and a way to give her something of me to keep when not with me.

Later that day, my wife saw me putting the bears into my car trunk—I planned on donating them elsewhere—and wondered whether I should keep them in case my patient should change her mind. Although certain she never would, I put the boxes away.

Almost a year later, Colleen asked if I still had the bears. When she heard that I did, she smiled but made it clear that she didn't want them. Not until many months later did she ask to see them, and only a year after that—following much therapy work around the bears, centering on their being abused and abandoned themselves—did she ask to take the mother bear home. As of this writing, the baby bear still sits in its box, "orphaned for being a very naughty bear" but safe with me.

Gift giving in reverse, though less common, presents a variation on the theme. A patient's need to give to us is one that needs to be confronted, though gently.

"Open it," Elisa ordered. I opened the child-wrapped gift and found a fancy card covered with hearts and I-love-you's. "Do you like it?" Elisa asked anxiously.

"You've given me so much," I replied. And she had, ever since we'd first met five weeks before. "Let's see. There was the bookmark and the mug. And then you gave me a lollipop and . . ." "Two other cards," Elisa interrupted. "And you made them all yourself. So much hard work," I said. "And for me!"

Elisa smiled with pleasure that I'd noticed all that she'd done.

Readers probably notice that I didn't reply with the expected and civil, "Yes, I like it very much." Why didn't I? Was I being cruel, I initially pondered, to deprive a sweet little girl of my approval, no less one trying to please me so hard? But feeling the compulsion of her giving counseled me otherwise. She was giving to me, it was clear, not because she loved me so much. How could she? She'd just met me. She gave because *she had to*. And that is why her gifts did not feel good in coming as much as they felt sad and frightened. But at that time Elisa herself didn't know for sure why she brought me presents. She learned why some weeks later when, having forgotten to pack her present from home, her mother reasonably refused to drive home to get it.

> Absolutely panicked and wanting desperately to make me a new gift right there on the spot, Elisa expressed her great fear that I'd be mad and not like her. Why wouldn't she? She had a father—divorced and living states away—who could explode over almost anything, including a well-meaning and homemade present?
> "You just want to make sure that I like you," I said.
> "Wouldn't you?" Elisa replied. Yes, I nodded back. I would.

An overadoring tenor and frequency of gifts can signal an idealized transference that needs attention. While the patient's valuing of us and treatment is generally favorable, it can lead to difficulties if unending in its intensity and duration. This is especially likely when children can't acknowledge any imperfections on our part yet find themselves extraordinarily critical of everyone else, even themselves, and whose life outside of therapy seems to be getting no better. A therapy full of nothing but love for the therapist is often rather empty and impotent.

I've seen other children whose regular gift giving was their way of asking me to give to them. In every instance my clarification of that wish has led to their no longer needing to give to me. And, of course, in the majority of instances when, feeling good about therapy, they bring us a card or a Christmas gift they made, children expect and deserve a normal, human thank you.

The giving of food, or snacks, is an even more common aspect of child therapy. For some clinicians the giving of snacks is automatic either because of clinic policy—all child patients, for example, get to visit the snack closet—or personal belief that feeding children is part of the natural adult relationship with children. They may judge their child patients to actually need the nutrition of an after-school snack to maintain their attention in the hour. Or, understandably, they may feel that this concrete feeding helps to relax the child or foster her good feelings toward the therapist and the work.

As one who occasionally but not routinely gives snacks, I find the giving of food to be one of those things we do at a particular time to give a particular child what she clinically needs, even if it's out of our usual therapeutic bounds.

> Nine-year-old Heather, orphaned early in her infancy, was brought to treatment because of her explosive temper.
>
> For months Heather showed me her finest moments, even stating, upon query, that she couldn't imagine anything I could do to get her angry the way so many other people seemed to do. Fortunately, this cheery prediction spoke more to the mounting resentment she feared would erupt even as she tried to suppress it. In plain English, she soon blew, big-time.
>
> After the rage passed, Heather began to experience a new feeling, an intense emptiness. She felt that she was a volcano that had spewed out everything inside, leaving a hollow cavity.
>
> "I'm hungry," Heather said in a little voice. She rubbed her stomach as might a toddler.
>
> "Would you like some cookies and milk?" I asked, deliberately using the words that so capture TLC. Heather nodded that she would. She devoured the snack in seconds, looking like a child who hadn't eaten for days.

For months after that session, Heather would ask for something to eat whenever she felt emotionally empty. She made it clear that physical hunger was an emptiness she could easily endure. It was a deeper sense of emptiness that was unbearable and that could be soothed somewhat by my feeding her. I'd been tempted to institute a weekly snack after that first one. But that would have diluted its specialness and dismissed her need. What would she do with a snack on days when she felt filled? What should she then do on days she felt inordinately hungry? What might she ask for when the cookies and milk that were always there no longer filled her?

I readily offer snacks to children who complain of their stomach aching from more pedestrian forms of hunger just as I typically offer a glass of water to the child who's thirsty or a hard candy to another whose throat is dry from talking or scratchy from a cold. I've brought out toast and fruit to a child (and his parents) who had to leave home without breakfast because of a power outage. And I've provided a weekly snack for children who've come from homes that grossly lack nurturing.

Much like the child who brings us gifts, we may encounter the child who brings two snacks—one for himself and one for us. Our response is best measured by what the child's gift intends as well as our own likes and needs.

> Maxwell slid a giant-sized soda and an even bigger bag of popcorn toward me while eating and drinking from his own. The third week in which he'd brought me food, I commented, "I wonder why you always bring me a snack." Maxwell casually explained that he felt rude eating in front of me. "When I bring food to stuff your face, I don't have to feel bad about stuffing mine."

Although this dynamic did not turn out to be a central one in Maxwell's work, our bite-sized discussion enabled him to come to therapy with just one snack, saving the teen some effort and money. This also proved to him, he told me, that I, his therapist, could handle his being straight with me, a belief that promoted his being straight with himself when facing other topics.

The reasons children bring us snacks are as varied as the colors of their jelly beans. A second child who brought me weekly snacks, for example, had a much larger agenda than Maxwell. Raised by a single and alcoholic father whom he helped to care for, he felt obligated to parent me, too. In a majority of cases I've found that it was the parents, not the child, who felt the need to bring a snack for me along with one for their child.

When children offer us the occasional snack, do we eat it? One simple answer: it depends on whether we want to. Intuitively, doesn't it seem best to take the child's offering with thanks, eating it with zest? Unfortunately, I find myself unable to do so. Sometimes I'm not hungry. Sometimes I don't like the snack. Sometimes I'm hungry and like the snack but am put off by the threads of Kleenex and pocket dust on the brownie, or I can't look past the just-up-the-nose or rear-end-scratching fingers that are handing me the cupcake. I've also learned the hard way never to eat foods that come from the hands of children with obvious colds and illness. It just isn't worth it.

When responding, we strive to see where the offer comes from. Responding either way to a no-big-deal kind of spur-of-the-moment offer is itself no big deal. The child hands us a stick of gum for no other reason than he's having one, has lots of them, and couldn't care less whether we take it. We are less nonchalant with children who appear or whom we know to care about the food they offer. Although I may not want to eat the opened string cheese that an isolated boy handed me—in his first positive overture toward me—I would not simply reject it but make clear his generosity and my appreciation. I hesitate to take food gifts with the implication that I'll eat them later unless they are something I'll truly eat. Otherwise, I set myself up for rejecting the child or having to lie—never therapeutically defensible—when next week he asks me how it tasted.

We frequently face our patients' requests for more involvement in their lives outside of treatment. They want us to buy Girl Scout cookies and raffle tickets and sponsor their walks for hunger. "Can you come to my baseball game?" they ask. "My school play is Friday night." Children naturally invite us to their homes to meet their pets, view their rooms, play their computer games, and eat dinner with their families. While these invites are usually qualified as needed opportunities to give me a chance to see their lives in the flesh—and in part they are—they express an unspoken longing that toddler patients express more openly. "Can you come live with me?"

What do we do with these requests? First, we must recognize that they are natural and to be expected. That they don't come more often is the bigger surprise and is probably evidence of children's somehow grasping that this relationship is different. Why wouldn't children ask that we underwrite their efforts to sell more popcorn than every other Boy Scout? If we are so interested in their lives, their requests imply, why wouldn't we want to do our share, if not everything we can, to assist them in winning the award for being the troop's best salesman?

The nature of the request, that is, how it is delivered and in what context, often guides our response.

Bursting into my office, Carl slammed three candy bars onto my desk. "You owe me three dollars," he stated. "Well, pay up, you stingy bastard." He pushed the bars into my lap, frustrated by the few seconds of my not replying.

"I know you want me to buy some candy," I said. "But I don't know anything else about it."

"Forget it," Carl snapped. He then took the candy bars, smashed them against the desk, and threw them into the wastebasket.

From the couch on which he now lay and cried, he continued his hard if failing sell. "Now you owe me six dollars."

"Six?"

"Three for the candy bars you ruined and three for the candy bars you have to buy."

"For the bars I ruined?"

"You're a bitch," Carl screamed. "Why couldn't you just give me the three dollars so I wouldn't have to get so mad?"

My continued and steady posture of mostly just listening led to a torrent of revelations of the ways in which Carl felt unheard. By the hour's end he was able to laugh at the way he'd accosted me while describing his hatred of selling things.

"I wish someone would just buy me that knife [the reward for selling a certain number of bars]." He told of his nervousness ringing neighbors' doorbells and having to explain what he was selling and why. "I feel like a little beggar," he said, making his hard-sell salesmanship understandable.

At the hour's end Carl apologized for blaming me as he salvaged the candy bars out of the basket. Sensing the sincerity in his sorry and having witnessed the hard work he'd done around the incident, I—above his insistence to the contrary—bought two of the candy bars. I held off from buying the third bar out of fear that my closing out the session too neatly would shut down the process that had just begun.

As we attend to the underlying motives in the child's asking for something, the right thing to do usually makes itself known, and we can generally accomplish a good deal of therapeutic work. When a girl asks me to attend her championship soccer game, my patient and empathic confirming of her pride and her wish to share it with me will probably give her most of what she wants. When the child's want persists, we try to be frank but caring. "I know you want me to see your room, but I don't visit the homes of children I work with." Such a candid reply, especially when we understand just how rejecting our decline can feel, tends to lead to good outcomes; in that case, the child spent weeks drawing me blueprints of the rooms in her house, plans that she verbally annotated with important feeling and insight.

There are times, however, when we may decide to do what the child asks with a minimum of exploration. For example, I readily bought a church raffle ticket from a developmentally disabled child who, through this activity, was bravely going out into the world in a new and assertive way. I promptly backed an extremely self-centered child's participating in a run for a battered women's shelter, the first time I'd ever seen him seem to care about another person or cause. Likewise, when a most caring girl asked me to donate an old stuffed animal to her collection for a disadvantaged children's Christmas program, I saw no need to examine her motivations.

We try to beware of urgent requests that we don't understand. Hey-buddy-can-you-spare-a-dime, incidentally tossed out in the hour's final minute, can be deceiving, however noble or harmless it may sound. Why, I wonder, did the child wait until now? My generally unmoving position that I cannot respond to something that is unclear to me even if it means missing some deadline, though frustrating, tends to strengthen the child's growing sense of trust and reliance on the therapy.

Children, being children, are built to test the limits and framework of therapy and their therapists. "Do I have to leave now?" (Yes, unless there are very good reasons not to, such as a psychologically compelling line of thought or discussion that warrants extending the hour.) "Can I leave early?" (No, unless it appears that you are truly ill, or there is some very special event that you should be on time to, or you've already done some very difficult work today working on issues of closeness and staying will overwhelm you, spoiling the session's progress.) "Can we go outside?" (With me, generally no, unless there is something you wish to show me on the outside, such as your dog who waits in the car.) Every aspect of the therapy that is clearly firm and sacred, the child will challenge to assess its integrity and ours.

"Have fun cleaning up," Lenice crowed at me as she headed for the door. A reckless eight-year-old who disrupted her home and classroom was now pushing my nose into her mess.

"You need to clean up," I calmly stated.

"What are you gonna do if I don't? Send me to bed without dinner? Tell my mother?"

Certain that I could not do the former and knowing from earlier discussions that I would not do the latter, Lenice had drawn the line boldly between the two of us. This was our battle.

"If you don't pick up the blocks, you won't get to use them next week," I replied.

"You wouldn't do that. Your job is to be nice to me."

"My job is to help you understand why you need to make a shambles everywhere you go."

Lenice smiled sheepishly, trying to look as if she could give a hoot, as she came back to clean up the room.

"Satisfied?" she asked provocatively as she kicked the last block across the floor.

"Lenice," I called to her in the waiting room. "You forgot one."

"You're a jerk," she muttered as she threw the one remaining block into the toy box before leaving with a slam of the door.

To have let Lenice off the hook would have played right into her delinquency-tempted hands. That she'd been coming to therapy for five weeks now suggested that she was ambivalent about her bad-girl lifestyle. Her testing me now underlined that suspicion. She was checking whether I could handle her. Could I, read the sequel, help her? My stubbornness concerning the last scrap of mess targeted her sociopathic streak. In the more wayward workings of her mind, were I to have overlooked that one measly block—what the heck, she cleaned up 99 percent of what she'd played with—she'd have beaten me, proving her badness and my unworthiness as the knight to tame her inner dragon.

If Lenice had been a well-meaning but disorganized child, I'd have helped her clean and said nothing about a block or two she'd missed. Were she a neurotic and overly self-critical child, I'd have said nothing, inside applauding her finally being able to make a mess without experiencing undue anxiety that I'd be mad or no longer like her.

To clean or not to clean is an issue that can take an even more complicated form.

> Tyler was an impulse-ridden, borderline 10-year-old who was still exquisitely vulnerable to stress from within and outside himself, though therapy had greatly decreased his susceptibility to psychotic regression. In recent months he'd come closer to acknowledging his frightful sense of himself as a worthless, perverted, and vile human being who deserved to die. This realization, while promising recovery, also threatened to do him in.
>
> "Blah, blah, blah," Tyler repeated in a crazed monotone meant to annoy me. But seeing little disturbance in me, Tyler raised the ante and the volume. "I'm going to relieve my anus on you," he dared, describing in great deal how he'd defecate on me and my office.
>
> Using the blocks, Tyler then built an elaborate outhouse in which he pretended to poop, this play contraption allowing him to exhibit his clothed rear end, relinquish (in fantasy) grown-up control over his bowels, and poop all over me all the while in the containment and displacement of a play toilet. A very neat, creative, and important piece of therapeutic work, it appeared to me.
>
> At the hour's end Tyler made one last noisy pretend bowel movement and walked to the door. "I'm not cleaning up," he said, teasing me but sounding ready to run back and clean up upon my expected demand that he do so.
>
> "You made mess all over my office, and you want me to clean it up?" I said with a smile.

Appreciating my good-natured acceptance—much in contrast with the harsher reactions he got from others in his life—he went to clean up on his own. But I gestured him away. "I'll be happy to clean your mess," I said. And I was.

Reading this account out of context could curl my own hair. How indulgent of me! Was I running the risk of inviting regression, leading a sick child to expect that he could find pleasure by relieving himself on me in his fantasy and play? Possibly, but Tyler's situation seemed to call for an exception in my usual framework.

Although coming in greater contact with his self-hatred—the basic precipitant of his self-destructive behavior and compulsion to repel those he seeks—he was not behaving worse. In his play he'd worked hard to create a wonderful play object, the toilet, in which to express his painful urges. My spontaneous willingness to clean up after him not only rewarded his good and higher-functioning play but also symbolically held him like the mother who still loves her not-yet-toilet-trained and poop-covered baby, even after the Tyler-baby shows her the aggression and hatred that he habitually uses to assault himself.

Child patients not only want more things from us, they often want more information about us. Do we have children? Wives? Pets? Were we happy children? Were we naughty? Did our parents love us? Did they die? Where is our mommy right now? The questions can be abstract. "What are your views of the universe and its meaning?" "Does your daddy punish you?" Although infinitely varied in their content and construction, these questions all seek to better know and understand us as our child patients attempt to better know and understand their own families and themselves.

How much do we tell? Once more, it depends on the child, the circumstances, and our own need to reveal or be private. Occasionally we encounter conscienceless and violent children whom we tell little about our personal lives mostly because we don't feel that we can trust them. But in circumstances in which we do not feel personally threatened by what children ask of us, we tend to examine their requests in terms of what makes clinical sense.

When our child patients ask if we have children, we look to know what they are asking. "Do you understand children?" "Do you know what it means to be a parent?" "Do you know what it means to love and care for a child?" "Do you let your children do things that my parents don't?"

"Are you stricter with your children than my parents are with me?" And, of course, the most painful, relevant, and seldom articulated worry of them all: *"Do you love your children more than you love me?"*

We have no difficulty grasping a child's wish to know us better. After all, we are privy—or at least work to make ourselves privy—to the deepest and most inner parts of our child patients' thoughts, feelings, and experiences. "Tell us more," we sometimes must appear to be saying, while we sit like two-dimensional dummies behind soundproof and bulletproof Plexiglas. "What about you?" the children wish to yell. "Never mind, tell me more. Tell me anything about your humiliations, your failures, and your defects." This is one reason why children are so eager to sit in our seats, take our positions, and play the head honcho, the therapist who probes us, their patients.

Often our deciphering the hidden question in their questions does the trick, allowing us to provide the comfort or confirmation they need. "You wonder if I ever got into trouble, if I know what it's like to feel like a screwup?" "You wonder if I've known hard times or if it all came easy to me?" "You worry that I must love my children more than you."

Sometimes, what children most want us to see is that the one-wayness of therapy feels unfair and frustrating. Children can ask personal questions motivated less by specific interest than a more generic need to get us to say something, anything about who we are. And as we all know, children can ask questions about us as a counteroffensive ploy to steer the discomforting spotlight away from themselves.

> "Got any kids?" "How old?" "Boys?" "Girls?" "They like sports?" "They get into trouble?" "You ever hit them?" With low-key efficiency, Gino asked me question after question. And I answered most of them.
>
> Knowing Gino and his family well from my work with a previous sibling, I didn't worry about sharing information with the 12-year-old. That he was interviewing me to ward off my doing the same to him was evident but not problematic. In his scrutiny of me, he more than revealed his own concerns as well as his prominent but long-denied wish to know his biological father, a man who had left the family when Gino was just a baby.

We all know moments when, in reply to a query or of our own accord, we deem it useful to disclose something personal that we hope will help a child patient.

"What would you know about crazy thoughts?" the pretend-pooping Tyler declared.

"We all have crazy thoughts."

"You mean even you wanted to poop everywhere when you were a baby?"

"Of course," I replied, assuming I must have.

"No kidding," he said, satisfied.

I've shared with certain children my educational mishaps, moments of social embarrassment, moments of fear, and moments of great disappointment. Partly because of their rarity, our disclosures can carry special meaning for our children patients. While overuse of disclosure can wear out quickly (the child doesn't listen or it comes across as a competition of childhoods), used sparingly and wisely, it can serve as a bridge to help children traverse especially hard experiences.

Although they may show interest in the facts themselves, any knowledge they glean about us tends to mean something. It is that meaning that we wish to see in order to help the therapy move as well as it can. When children learn that I have children, I want to know what that means to them and watch how they deal with it. "You're married," a young girl announces, just now seeming to notice my ring, though in her fourth month of treatment. "So what about it?" goes my gut reaction, a curiosity that, while not verbalized, leads to my observing and interacting around this issue for many hours to come.

Probably the most controversial and touchiest of framework strains is the child's (or therapist's) wish to give or take physical affection. To want to touch, pat, hold, hug, and kiss those we love goes without saying. That children want to do these things to us could not make more sense. If we show them all of the caring and respect to earn their most genuine trust and love, why would they not want to feel physically closer to us?

Leaving the obvious legal and ethical considerations to other books, let's focus on the clinical. To exaggerate the importance of the legal, subsumed by the clinician's self-interest, can cause us to misperceive clinical needs that run no risk of violating any child's trust or boundaries.

When a child suddenly and rarely shows us some affection—a quick and fleeting hug, leaning against us when showing us their wonderfully improved grades—it would be amiss, I think, to push the child away, as it would also be to pick the child up in our arms to prolong and deepen the embrace. We would calmly and comfortably, it is hoped, allow the child his expression, equally allowing him to retreat and go on with therapy, processing that physical contact only as he and the therapy judged to be necessary.

However, should a child want regular physical contact, we exercise a different kind of judgment, setting a limit with empathic caring for the child's likely feelings of rejection as well as inviting exploration of the longing that moved the child to ask for our physical show of love.

"Do you care about me?" the bright six-year-old Nellie asked, standing beside me.

"Yes."

"Do you *really* care about me?" she persisted.

I nodded that I did.

"Then how come you don't let me sit in your lap?" Nellie asked, her smiling face turning serious, her hand holding on to my knee.

That was a question I've faced with dozens of children. Sitting on the lap of the adults whom they love is part and parcel of their lives. It is the place they go for help, to be read to, to be told a story, and to be held.

"You want to sit up here so badly. I know that."

"Then why can't I?"

And why can't she? What's wrong with therapists showing their child patients that kind of caring? We often feel real love for our patients, so why not show it in real and concrete terms that a child can feel and understand?

"I don't allow the children I see to sit on my lap," I said softly but firmly.

"Oh," she said, still standing aside me, having pulled her hand off my leg to the chair's armrest.

I wanted my statement to make clear that it was my decision. "I can't allow children to sit on my lap" would be a bit of a lie, placing the blame on an outside authority, an agent Nellie would have been powerless to rile against. "Children don't sit on their therapists' lap" might be largely true, but it too would beg the question and push the responsibility away from me and the therapy. "It's not right for children to sit on their therapist's lap" would be worse, turning the child's reasonable and healthy request on its ears, suggesting now that she is somehow a bad girl for desiring that.

"My grandfather let me," Nellie told me sadly.
"You miss him," I said, feeling no need to turn away the little hand that had come back to rest on my own.

Every child's wish to sit on our lap or to be given affection in any other way asks for love and security in its own unique fashion. Nellie's request revealed the longing for a beloved and recently deceased grandfather, one who, I'd been told, had loved her devotedly and well. Nellie didn't need my lap, a lap that would soon no longer be in her life. She needed my help in grieving a grandfather, doing so, moreover, as she had a mother who could not accept either her father's death or her own and her daughter's mourning.

In the once-in-a-while instances when a child, experiencing an epiphanal moment of pain or joy, clinically demands some affection, I would not push the child away; instead, I'd permit the hug to come and go on its own. However, we are cautious about giving such affections on a more frequent basis, knowing that doing so may be confusing and may keep the child from doing the more important therapeutic work concerning the wish or need for hugs and kisses.

Some would argue that younger children need that kind of love. But it isn't true that such love is best coming from their therapists. And the argument that they are young is no argument at all. Younger children, particularly those who've been abused or come from seductive homes, can be just as confused by affection and physical attention. That argument also evokes a bigger question: At what age then would you pull back the hugs? Might a therapist hug a six-year-old boy but push him away on his seventh birthday? If such dilemmas confuse us, imagine what they do to the child, especially to one whose experiences have made him vulnerable.

Even when we set the limit, however, we are careful to protect the longing and esteem of the child we've rejected. "I won't be hugging you," I've told more than one child with Down syndrome—children whom the love of people has made extremely susceptible to exploitation—"but our hands can hug" (in a good handshake). While disliking my not giving them back a hug and feeling much cooler about a handshake, these children have learned not only how to feel the love they want through my hand but how to deal more age appropriately with others, to get more worthwhile attention, while minimizing the danger in their trusting social interactions.

And in times of physical pain, I don't hesitate to do what I can. When Ethan's babysitter dropped him off at my office feeling sick and with his head cut, I did not need to question my prompt attention to providing first aid and comfort. I open windows and turn up the heat readily to keep my patients comfortable. For the children who, to my continued amazement, brave their way to therapy even when ill, I think nothing of tucking the office blanket over them or turning down the lights to soften their migraine. These children remind us palpably that there are many doable and safe ways to let our child patients know that we care.

The reasons we therapists break the rules are many. We may wish to please our patients so they will be happier, so they will like us, or so they will not be angry. Some clinicians might feel the press to please their patients so they will keep coming, keep on as bill-paying customers. We also act out of unconscious pulls. Only by asking ourselves over and over, "Why am I being different with this child at this time?" can we ensure that we act out of clinical rightness and not to gratify or protect ourselves. Clinicians who truly intervene for their patient's best interests, not for self-serving rationalizations, are in little danger of behaving illegally or unethically.

Like the wondrous jazz musician who must first master the basics in all their complexity or the schoolteacher who must establish her authority before she can ease the class into a happier and more self-controlled place, we must build our therapies on strong and dependable frameworks. Indeed, we can't afford to do otherwise. Ignoring the framework will nearly always lead to erratic, unreliable, and weak—if not abusive or dangerous—therapy experiences. Embracing it too rigidly, however, without room for necessary adaptions to the child's fluctuating needs, will forsake some of the most golden opportunities for therapeutic intervention and growth. We must remind ourselves that there are no absolute right or wrong answers. The right answers we seek are much more complex, variable, and changeable.

Part III

The Rest

11

Handle with Care: Working with Parents

One of the most important truths of our work is also one of the most obvious: without a child, there can be no child therapy. For the majority, it is parents or other caregivers who arrange for and bring children to our doorstep. Moreover, once a treatment is underway, its outcome hangs at least as much on what the parents do as it does on what transpires in the therapy office. Knowing so much is at stake, how can we best meet and enlist parents in our joint mission of helping them to help their children?

Perhaps the place to begin is to recognize that bringing one's child for therapy is generally a courageous and loving act. Entrusting our children to a kindergarten teacher, with all her familiarity, accountability, and public exposure, is hard enough. We can easily imagine how much more difficult and threatening it is to bring our children to someone who will meet with them in private to tamper with their minds and souls, while they along the way will likely reveal and confront our darkest and most regretted parenting moments. Yet this is sometimes forgotten when we find ourselves in conflict with parents or when we are feeling critical of ways they treat our patients, their children.

We convey our understanding of this challenge by offering a compassionate and open ear to parents' stories and to what they have to say about their children and by respecting their life choices. Although these choices may not be the same ones we would make or even in their children's best interests, they are their own and for that reason alone need to be accepted and understood. Until parents feel that we care about the reasons they have gotten to where they are or how they've lived, they won't be open to changing their ways, particularly to the ways that others, such as ourselves, have in mind.

We try to be honest. Honest about what we will be doing, honest about what we can and can't do. We present ourselves honestly, not just in terms of experience, training, and credentials but with regard to our motives and perspective. If we are asked things we don't know, we say so. But when we do know things that need to be said, we say them, even when they're difficult. Despite their protests, I have met few parents or children who aren't willing to hear the truth if it's offered with respect, concern, and in the context of some hope—hope in the form of promising strategies or resources, however dismal the situation.

Through this combination of empathy, respect, and honesty, we begin to build an alliance with the parents much like the one we build with our child patients. This growing relationship will serve many critical functions in the course of the child's treatment. Parents will feel good and trust us enough to enter their family to work with their child; they'll also feel sufficiently okay with spending their time, money, and hope on what we might do for them. As the relationship develops further, the growth of trust and mutual understanding will offset our inevitable misunderstandings or mistakes so that parents won't be as quick to pull the plug on treatment or undermine it indirectly.

This increasing well of positive feeling allows parents to reveal themselves with corresponding candor. Their sensing that we don't see them as such awful parents ironically enables them to share and process the sometimes awful acts for which they feel ashamed or guilt-ridden. "That's nothing," many parents have indicated after mildly losing control with their children in my presence. "You should see me when I've really lost it." More times than not, parents speak these words, not after I've put down what they did or insinuated that things must be worse at home but after I've noted how much they dislike their own behavior or have waited for their own reactions. The liking and respect that parents feel for us, returning that which we give them, also becomes leverage that we'll surely need at times in therapy. In tougher therapeutic times, for example, when confronting even bigger, badder, or more painful circumstances and attitudes, we'll draw on that accumulated positive relationship, like a rainy-day account, to neutralize the hurt and rupturing influence of our interventions.

The dedication we share with parents to work on the child's behalf also provides a channel of communication for information. What is the problem? How precisely does it show itself at home, in school, and on the playground? When did it begin? What is the atmosphere at home like? Has there been abuse, neglect, or less startling trauma? How does bedtime go? Why did previous therapies work or fail? Parents can give us the data we need on current circumstances, family history, development, and every aspect of their child's life and background.

The importance of parents' filling us in applies not just to the evaluation phase but throughout the treatment. There are unusual children who are able and willing to talk about the matters that most trouble them and others; most children try to avoid these areas for as long as they can. The notion of children blossoming in the safe and nurturing arms of therapy is a lovely one, but most children, like most grown people, tend to turn away from painful and difficult parts of their lives unless somehow pushed or otherwise motivated. If it were not for parents telling me, I might never know that a child has been failing three subjects, lighting fires, talking of suicide, or experiencing countless other problems that require my attention in therapy.

Parents often need training, particularly early in a treatment, to know how to best keep us informed. Although the material they give us early on is important, it's the week-by-week updates that can alert us to relevant events and reactions in the child's life.

"Anything I should know?" I often ask casually of the parent who's taken a seat in the waiting room. Parents learn that by *anything* I mean whatever concerns them, needs to be known, or might facilitate the day's therapy. It's here that parents tell me of upcoming doctor visits that their child is obsessing over, increased aggression or sibling rivalry at home, calls from school, or the child's uncharacteristic attempt to avoid coming to the session that day. This information can frankly give meaning to a stale hour, particularly as children are prone to avoid matters they're trying not to feel or think about. Most parents quickly learn how to use this space around a child's hour to communicate efficiently.

I similarly invite or urge parents to use my answering machine to leave bulletins reporting an upsetting moment, a good example of a current problem, or a troubling passing comment (e.g., "I'm never going to amount to anything!"). Don't worry, I say, about leaving an extensive or elegant message, "just blurt out what's happening." Parents become skilled at telling us what we need to know. Knowing this route is open to them makes parents a bit more observant of their child and themselves and results in better parenting. This arrangement may sound onerous to the clinician, but it actually eases our work and allows us to help children and their parents more quickly and clearly.

But getting information on the sly from parents raises its own issues. I make clear to my child patients that I want their parents to keep me informed. Most children don't mind. Parents may cringe to learn that I openly let their children know of our communications, but they soon learn that it isn't traumatic. Having our contact out in the open allows us to bring up topics directly. "I heard about your dog [dying]." "You know your mom told me about the suspension on Friday." More times than not, we don't need to make specific mention of what we learn. Our simply knowing gives us a context in which to decipher what the child says and plays in the session.

Parents also gain finesse at bringing up matters in a way that moves a child's work along, especially around small but critical junctures. They learn to catch our eye or ask if we think it advisable that they tell us something. "Do you think it makes sense to just come in for a few moments?" I'll ask. When parents think it does, they usually have good reasons. These mini child–parent sessions, occasionally expanding to an hour but more routinely lasting minutes, can propel some of the deepest and most difficult work we do with the child.

Unsurprisingly, there are times and parents that require a variation on this theme of access. Some parents never call and share little information around their child's hour, letting us know at their meetings and only after too much time and to our enormous frustration that things are no better or worse than ever, moving us to invoke a communication initiative a bit more forcefully. Other parents need our influence in the other direction.

> "He screamed at me all morning. He didn't clean up his room when I asked him to. And," she added, as her son, Carlos, sat across from me, quietly listening, "he's been walking around the house with a major attitude." When she left the office, I looked at Carlos, my eyes asking him what he thought of all his mother had said. Just as he began to tell me, with an abrupt knock and sudden opening of the door, she stuck her head back through the door. "Oh, and I'm not sure we like some of the kids he's been hanging around with either."
>
> After she left again, Carlos rolled his eyes. "She always does this," he said. "She talks about me to anyone who'll listen." Carlos described how his mother habitually gave detailed reports of his misbehaviors to his father, her friends, and his grandparents. "I understand why she gets upset sometimes," he explained, "but does she have to tell the whole world about it?"

Carlos's mother meant well, but she meant other things, too. When she wasn't filling me in on her son's failings, she was reporting on those of her husband and her aging parents.

Carlos's mother felt let down by almost all of the important people in her life. Once I made clear my understanding of this—which I did outside of her son's presence, at an hour's end after he'd run to the car—I could ask her how it must feel for her son to hear her speak so harshly of him in front of me. She easily grasped my message. This question of family dynamics continued to be one that we worked on in parent meetings. Why did she need to put her son and others down so much? In the meantime she came up with more constructive means of sharing useful information with me.

Parents, particularly early in treatment, tend to see our communicating as intended to convey the dirt, the ways in which their child's or their own behavior has gone awry. Gradually, often with our help, they come to also see the value of sharing good news: a markedly improved report card or disappearance of a nasty behavior. But it is more important that parents be led to report the teeny steps that over time amount to therapeutic progress.

> "Things were okay," Mr. Toyo replied dismissively in response to my asking how their Sunday family day had been. "But when we returned the canoes," he continued, his voice growing louder, "Kyle just lost it. Sara was handing Kyle their paddles, and—"

"Kyle went canoeing?" I interrupted to ask, having heard so many times about his utter dread and rejection of the very water sports his father loved.

"Yeah," Mr. Toyo answered, seeming to be caught momentarily by what he'd failed to notice, "but it was just a shallow lake. It wasn't as if we sailed out in the ocean."

I was tempted to pounce on that, to point out Mr. Toyo's impossible demands of his son, but the slight hesitation caused me to wait.

"Actually, that must have been a pretty big thing for Kyle, don't you think?" Mr. Toyo asked.

I nodded my agreement.

"But anyway, when Sara handed Kyle their paddles—"

"*Their* paddles?" I asked, again cutting him off.

"Yeah, they shared a canoe."

I looked Mr. Toyo in the eyes, and he immediately caught my drift. "They don't usually do things together, do they?"

I smiled.

"Maybe the day was better than I recognized."

Getting it, Mr. Toyo was then able to describe what he'd originally wished to, his continuing frustration with Kyle's behavior. My gently urging him to see the little giant steps that Kyle had taken buoyed Mr. Toyo; warned him of the ways in which he, always so aware of his son's shortcomings, failed to notice his achievements; and led to his giving Kyle more praise and credit for such shows of bravery and change. Not surprisingly, this modest discussion began Mr. Toyo's own exploration of the ways in which he acted as critical and unimpressible as his own father had. Encouraging parents to share these miniature victories can foster their being more attentive and observant of their child's efforts and accomplishments, give them week-by-week encouragement as they wait for the larger therapeutic rewards, and make them more aware and proud of their own parenting steps forward.

The information hotline that runs between the therapist and parents accomplishes even more. Establishing this line helps to make parents feel held when they are not in our offices or waiting rooms. It helps parents feel less alone with their troubles, reduces the likelihood that they will somehow sabotage or undo therapy due to frustration and resistance, facilitates their positively attaching to us, and lends them ego support for withstanding the stresses of their home lives.

We establish this communication, this relationship, with parents in the service of achieving therapeutic goals with their children, our primary patients. For many, parenting well is not as natural a process as some would like us to think. One of our chief objectives is for the parents to come to appreciate where the child is and what she needs from many different aspects.

Where is the child developmentally? For example, what is the developmental meaning of a child who often cries for her pacifier? If the child is one-year-old, it is as it should be. If the child is three years old and otherwise quite normal, we may together discover that her not wanting to give up her nucky has intensified since beginning preschool. Regressing at the age of five years and crying for the pacifier she spontaneously gave up at age two could relate to the recent birth of a baby brother. An eight-year-old's buying herself a pacifier and using it secretly may be giving a message to parents who, fearful of overdependence, forcibly weaned her of all sucking early in the first year. And while interest in the pacifier can signal an untoward reaction to stress in a well-loved child, it can be a sign of growth, of openness to attachment and nurturance, in a neglected and hardened child.

Seeing the developmental context of the child, particularly that in which troubling symptoms or behaviors occur, is critical in determining what we should do. We reassure the young parents who worry, making clear that their instinct to allow their baby to suck all she wants is a good one. We help the three-year-old and her parents cope with her separating to preschool, a decision about which the parents felt ambivalent, even guilty. We play with the five-year-old who, having a good home and able parents, must grieve the changes that having a sibling brings, helping her parents to see her regression as something natural, not to be squelched and that will pass. Deeply understanding the feeling that drove the eight-year-old to buy her own pacifier, we help her to better understand her dependency and oral needs as well as the hurt inflicted by her parents' well-intentioned deprivation, just as we work with her parents to see the reasons they have such reservations and discomfort about nurturing their child. With the loved child who is regressing, we take her stress seriously, working to resolve it externally as well as to enable her to withstand it better. But for the child who has nearly given up on humanity, we may do little more than celebrate and nurture his allowing himself the pleasure of a good suck.

Helping parents to know where their child is intellectually, emotionally, socially, and the rest and how the reasons for referral fit into that picture implicitly helps them to understand what we do or don't do in treatment. That knowledge, like most, will take some of the mysterious fear out of their relationship with their child, giving them data from which they can now make informed and more effective choices. It may propel parents to become active in ways long overdue (e.g., raising expectations for the child) or to chill out (e.g., not assess every moment of the child's life), making more comfortable space for their child to be and grow. What parents come to learn can alleviate worry and remorse, as when they realize that their child's state is a transitional and natural developmental phase. It can also be quite painful, as when a father comes to see how his limitations and misparenting have caused his child hurt and hardship.

Closely tied to development is the question of temperament. If developmental research has taught us anything, it is that children are all born different. Some infants are bold, some timid, some curious, some active, some passive, some affable, some cranky, some stoic, some sensitive. Infants, temperamentally speaking, come in all shapes and sizes. Part of our role as child therapists is to help parents recognize and accept who their child is temperamentally. We can't wholly reverse a child's development, nor should we. But how parents' temperaments interact with their children's does have great effect.

If I learn that a boy is quite shy, for example, I can help parents recognize that they unduly push him into situations that overwhelm him or make him feel less loved and worthy than his older sister who so easily takes center stage. Conversely, I sometimes recommend strategies to help parents respond to their child's temperament, showing how that same child might benefit from gentle urging to pursue activities or not to be treated with such kid gloves.

Issues of the child's temperament often connect directly with issues of a parent's temperament.

"I don't know what to do with him anymore." Mrs. Ellsworth spoke confidently and with disgust. Her nine-year-old Sam stood at the window, looking outward. "It was his birthday, and he barely had fun. All of the other children were screaming and running around the house, having a complete blast."

"Eric wasn't," Sam interjected. "He was—"

But his mother interrupted. "Eric was up and down the tree house at least a dozen times when he wasn't diving in the pool. Does he take diving lessons?" Mrs. Ellsworth asked, seeming to forget her irritation for the moment.

Sam said nothing.

"I sign you up for tennis, soccer, kayaking, but it never grabs you." Then she spoke to me, as if delivering her case to the judge and expecting me to affirm her disapproval. "All Sam wants to do is read and do whatever it is he does out in the yard."

"You sign me up for activities you want me to do, not things I like. You wanted a great athlete for a son, someone you can ski with on weekends and show off at the club. Well, I know you're disappointed, but I'm not that son. And what I do outside is not whatever. I study nature and wildlife."

"He's obsessed with drawing pictures of mushrooms and flowers."

"Is he good at it?" I asked her.

Seeing his mother lost for an answer, Sam chimed in. "She's never looked at them."

Sam was quite right. His mother, a fine athlete, had wanted a son to share her love of sports. She envied the mothers of the confident boys who played golf and tennis at their country club. Her son's preference for quiet and intellectual pursuit repelled her. While our work together didn't change the basic nature of either Sam or his mother, it helped her to see how his being so different from her frustrated and upset her and led to her misparenting him.

Such mismatches in temperament are common. Bold parents who dislike their child's quietness. Inhibited parents who don't know where that exhibitionist of a son came from. Fearful parents whose brave children hold their hands at the doctor's or who provocatively drag them to the roller coaster. Discovering how their own temperaments affect their perception of their child's can make a difference. It reduces parents' bewilderment and dislike of who their child is as well as the risk that they will intervene in ways that either ignore the child's potential for growth or push him to climb cliffs beyond his capacities or wishes.

Although we tend to encounter families only after the child is several years old, their asynchronies in temperament start impacting on them from birth. A mother able to wholly console and nurture her firstborn may find her extremely active and irritable second child much too much, his edgy personality so at odds with her own. Day by day, the frustration that results at either end of the relationship can lead to major misparenting and hurt for both parent and child. Coming to understand the tension of that mismatch at a later stage of childhood can prove helpful and reparative, even though the truth hurts.

While some referring problems reflect innate aspects of the child's functioning (anxiety or learning problems based mostly, if not completely, on neurobiology), others originate out of psychodynamics. As the therapy unravels these dynamics and illustrates dysfunctional patterns, we enlighten parents about what their child's symptoms or misbehaviors mean, what psychological functions they serve, for the child as an individual or the family as a whole.

> Scott was a sixth grader with an intelligence solidly above average. Yet he had been doing increasingly poorly over the academic year, receiving four Ds on his last report card. His teacher observed that he "had to work hard" to do so poorly, knowing that even the most minimal effort and cooperation would have brought higher grades to a boy as bright as he. Scott's deteriorating grades greatly distressed his parents, both of whom had professional degrees.

Over months of therapy, Scott came to understand that he had indeed unconsciously worked hard to not do well. His not handing in homework, not listening to assignments or instruction, and not paying attention to what he read were not motivated by an inherent neurological or learning disorder; Scott simply resented his parents' exaggerated and singular investment in academic achievement.

His parents, preoccupied with their work, had little time for him, and when they did, they used it to scrutinize his school performance. There was little fun in the house—no television, no sports; reading was designated as the home's official outlet for relaxation. Learning left Scott feeling cold and empty, burdened with the need to achieve and lacking good feeling, particularly when he compared what went on at friends' livelier, less intellectual homes with what happened in his own.

Our deciphering the good reasons for Scott's hostility toward school and learning enabled him to make better, less self-spiting decisions on his own behalf. Of equal import, my clarifying Scott's behavior for his parents moved them to examine themselves, their parenting, and their relationship to their work. Their confirmation that his feelings were justified—that they ignored him and much of life in favor of their work—freed up Scott to express his intellectual potential as he saw fit.

Just as we strive to demystify our child patients' anxiety, pessimism, suspicion, mistrust, fear, and shame for both them and their parents' edification, we try to clarify the sources of their small behaviors. "Matt snapped at you [his father] because he felt belittled by your laughing [when he tried, with pride, to tell of the ways he helped you work in the yard over the weekend]." "Ivy isn't talking with me because she believes you [her mother] will be hurt if she complains about you [in therapy]." "Caitlin [a supreme worrier] hasn't been eating the past few days on account of hearing a news report about tainted food poisonings."

Our disclosing what's behind their child's behavior or symptoms holds much utilitarian value for parents. Discovering the psychological functions these behaviors serve can minimize parents' taking it all personally. Their child, they grasp, does this or that, not mostly to irritate or oppose them but to protect her own psyche, to make her life bearable and doable. Unchained from their retaliative imperatives, they may find themselves more able and willing to parent in ways that promote their child on her self-directed recovery.

A counterpoint to helping parents understand their children's motives is helping them uncover their own.

"I don't care what you do, just fix him," Dr. Jamison said to me, meaning it. He referred to his nine-year-old son, Zachary, a hellion on two legs. Zack was everything his 66-year-old father was not. Dr. Jamison, a professor of history, was highly cerebral, unathletic, and deliberate in his motion. Although bright, Zack had little interest in books, much preferring to be in action of almost any kind, as long as it was high speed and fun.

Our work soon came to focus on Dr. Jamison, a reluctant father who was more than satisfied with having raised three grown children from two previous marriages. He had brought Zack to me with a mandate to calm him down quickly, using drugs if necessary, but Dr. Jamison also confessed, with not much coaxing, his worry of growing older, noting how Zack's boyish enthusiasm and energy made him feel that much older and slower. It also brought to the forefront Dr. Jamison's regret that he'd not been there for any of his children and his awareness that he was much more at home with books and ideas than with real people, even people he loved. He acknowledged that he'd never been a robust person, even as a boy, and that his whole life he'd harbored envy for those pursuing a vigorous existence.

These insights led to Dr. Jamison's growing less critical of Zack's healthy robustness and to a rapidly growing mutual interest in each other's lives, Dr. Jamison cheering Zack on athletically and Zack beginning to hang around his father's reading room.

There is much therapeutic reward in advancing parents' awareness of what they really think and feel about themselves, their child, and their parenting. But this work is fraught with pain and regret. We all want to believe that we hold nothing but good feeling and thoughts for our children. Confessing one's hatred toward a child is a hard thing to do. Likewise, admitting their own fears of separation or their jealousy or envy for their child does not come easily.[1]

Therapists aspire, moreover, to reveal how what parents do sometimes serves to protect their own esteem or tries to repair and compensate for hurts and neglects in their own childhoods or adult lives. Our work with parents in this regard typically runs slowly and carefully. Rather than hammer parents on the head with instances of their misperceptions and misparenting, we—by listening, being safe, and intervening aptly—seek to create the atmosphere and right amount of tension that leads parents to confront themselves. Instead of blasting and shaming them, we attempt to hold them as they whip themselves, keeping them afloat and hopeful even as they feel themselves sinking under the weight of their anguished revelations. (This latter part shouldn't be unduly hard for us, for however gloomy and self-hating their words, it is almost always encouraging when parents own up to their misparenting.)

Associated with the goal of parents' knowing themselves better is that of fostering their interest in and capacity for taking their child's perspective. Sometimes we foster this by extrapolating to the parent's adult life. "Imagine what it would feel like," I said to one father, "if your wife came home one day and said, all excited, 'Honey, guess what? I so enjoy loving you that I've brought home a second husband so we can be an even happier family.'" This analogy, heavy-handed and probably overused as it was, moved this father beyond his intolerance for his daughter's regressed reaction to the birth of a new sister. To make the child's situation and feelings more vivid for a parent, drawing comparisons between school and the workplace, adult ideals and childhood dreams, and the parent's and child's childhoods (i.e., intergenerational dynamics) can work wonders.

Unfortunately, some parents are just so far from their child's world (or so defended) that our work needs to be less ambitious. "I know it's hard to understand how Timmy can be so afraid of the school bus," I gently said to one father, conveying that I understood his frustration. "But he is afraid, very afraid, so what can we do to help him grow braver?" Timmy's father was not ready to examine his own counterphobic daredevilry and how it affected his son; he was prepared, though, to work constructively on helping his son overcome his fears.

Implicit in the goal of parents' taking their child's perspective is their taking seriously the impact that their own behaviors, words, and demeanor have on their child. Most parents take for granted the ways they parent, even ways that may be harmful or waste energy and time. And so we carefully cite their behavior or demeanor. "Is Shawna the only one in the family who's quick to criticize?" I ask of parents I know to be critical. Similarly, we urge parents to consider the effect on their child of their passivity, their impulsivity, or their always needing to be right.

Some of this work occurs in the transferencelike relationship that evolves between parent and therapist. "What's it like for you to see my family?" I asked one mother who could not understand her daughter's envy of my children. My query evoked the mother's saddened fantasy that her family would never be as joyous and loving as she imagined mine to be. In another instance a father complained, "My son's so unable to take criticism," only minutes before he himself had felt insulted by a remark of mine. When we noted the connection, this father discovered links between his own narcissistic vulnerability and his son's.

As therapists, we hope that seeing the influence of their misparenting will deter parents. Yet many, even after realizing its effects, continue their marital battling, drinking, or other serious indulgences. In such cases we work toward preventing parents' punishing their children doubly by adding the burden of secondary blame to the original behavior. Growing up with alcoholic parents, for example, is beyond horrid, but it is even more horrid when those parents blame their child for their drinking or deny the reality the child sees accurately and maybe complains of.

As child therapists we of course do much parent guidance. We educate parents about what children of that age, ilk, gender, circumstance, and so forth are like. We help them to see their child's need for love and discipline, and we provide instruction on limits and consistency. We try to reduce stress and introduce methods to cope with the stress that can't be avoided. We offer reassurance when we can do so honestly, and we hold parents' hands when they are frightened and shaky.

We offer all the help we possibly can so that parents can create a home atmosphere most conducive to the child's progress in therapy. Parents who put out the money and effort to bring their child to us generally want to help bring about therapeutic gains. And we don't mind giving bits of advice, together with our big explanations of what is going on, to move things along in the family or remove roadblocks to the child's healthful momentum. To that end we prepare parents for what might happen. Such predictions can take the edge off potentially noxious behavior.

> "Lorrie may become a lot more outspoken and ornery as he grows less inhibited," I warn, using interesting adjectives that connote something more intriguing than might the words *rude* and *crude*. And Lorrie sure did. But anticipating this obnoxious change helped Lorrie's parents to understand it as growth on the road toward greater confidence. Quietly encouraged by it, they didn't need to punish Lorrie or even make much noise about his.

Putting a child's change into a therapeutic and developmental context, provided that it belongs there, can provide parents the support, inspiration, and principles they need to make room for their child's growth. Such explanations go miles toward preventing them from making well-intentioned attempts to stop tears, tantrums, outbursts, and withdrawal, any or all of which might be temporarily necessary to the child's ongoing development.

Throughout this work with parents, we show them how we and therapy work. We keep our doors open, welcome their input and observations, and respect their undeniable sovereignty as the parents who love their child best of all. Rather than merely tell them what we do (though that can have its place), we demonstrate it in the office, in the waiting room, on the phone, and in between. Ever remembering how bad bringing one's child to therapy can make parents feel, we try to bring insights or make recommendations as subtly and nonthreateningly as we can. We watch for signs of narcissistic injury and encourage parents to share with us frustrations and anger that we have caused them. Whatever we think of our helpfulness and skill, we make clear that it is the parents' privilege, if not obligation, to alert us to their disappointment or disapproval of what we and therapy are doing or not doing.

In short, moment by moment, incident by incident, misunderstanding by misunderstanding, and session by session, our connection with parents builds, slowly but steadily, growing ever stronger and more effective through to our final hour with them and their child.[2]

NOTES

1. Oberschneider (2002) offers a readable historical and clinical look at transference in parent guidance.

2. Readers are referred to Ack, Beale, and Ware (1975); Arnold (1978); Chethik (1976); Colm (1964); Dawley (1939); Novick and Novick (2005); and Sperling (1994) for traditional and wise views on parent guidance. Siskind's (1997) more recent book on working with parents is thorough and instructive.

12

Handle with Care, Part II: More Work with Parents

Now that we've spotlighted general aspects of parent guidance, it's time to explore some specific and challenging situations that commonly arise in that work. Child therapists learn fast that they treat not just a child but parents too, one to four of them, parents who can be supportive or hostile, understanding or dense, loving or hating (it's true), trusting or paranoid, parents who can be just about anything, including those who don't agree in any way with the other parents who may be involved in a child's treatment and life. When in our work with parents, do we wear kid gloves or those made of soft fleece? When do we need wrist supporters for heavy lifting and exerting pressure? And when do we put on boxing gloves, meaning when, if ever, do we take off our listening caps and get firm and tough?

A good place to begin our study is with the reluctant parent, the mother or father who is skeptical of child therapy. When we think about what bringing a child for therapy can mean to parents, we can understand and hear their reservations. Some parents will bring their doubts right to us. They'll question our credentials and training, bully our intellects with their own, ask tough questions, and debate what we say. We try our best to be nondefensive. It's not always easy, especially when we are starting out or early in our career. We strive to answer directly.

"Fair question. I went to Boston College where I got a degree in counseling." "It's clear that you're very bright, and you wonder whether I'm smart enough to understand your gifted daughter." "Yes, you're right. I am young, and I realize that I look even younger than my age." "This is my third year working with children and their families." "I am a graduate student and trainee. An experienced and senior supervisor oversees my work here at this clinic." "I could give you a bunch of reasons why your son needs therapy, but it's more important that I grasp your reasons for knowing why he doesn't." Nothing disarms an attack and wins over "enemies" more than taking their questions seriously. They may doubt or fear our competence and motives, but they can't help but feel heard and impressed by our mature willingness to withstand their scrutiny. Sometimes, parents reveal their misgivings more passively.

We were through our initial parent meeting, and Evan's father had barely spoken. Even when I'd steered questions his way—"I'm really interested in *your* take of what's going on with Evan?—he ducked, looking to his wife or shrugging his shoulders. For most of the hour and despite his few words, however, he managed to tell me a lot. While his wife and I spoke, he played with his cuticles, fiddled with his PDA, studied his watch, and sometimes rolled his eyes.

"You okay with this?" I asked him.

"Me?" he replied, as if it could be anyone else. "Yeah, don't mind me, I'm fine with anything *she wants*."

"What I want?" his wife shot back. "Our son tried to hang himself. He was in a hospital. They told us he needs to talk to somebody."

"You don't have to like being here," I said casually. "A lot of good people disagree with this whole business."

"Yeah, well I guess I'm one of them. No offense or anything, you seem like an all right guy. But I got to tell you, we had a pretty bad experience at the hospital. They pretty much said"— Sudden emotion choked Evan's father, his eyes welled, he took a deep breath. "They pretty much said we made him want to kill himself."

"They said that?" I asked quietly. Both parents nodded. "No wonder you're not sure about this," I replied. "And me."

"I've just being waiting for you to lower the boom," Evan's father said.

"And accuse you of making Evan want to die?" I asked.

Evan's father hung his head.

If we too vigorously provoke or challenge parents when they oppose us, we risk getting off to a very bad start and turning a molehill into something much bigger and harder to surmount. I try to remind myself that parental resistance is probably not aimed at me personally as much as it expresses important and well-founded apprehension. More times than not, one or two accepting comments can put parents' good reasons on the table and start making headway beyond their apprehension toward a working alliance. As readers can see, it didn't take much to convince Evan's father to surrender to his deeper wish that his son and family get the help they needed. If I'd taken offense, avoided the issue, or dug my heels in, we might have gotten stuck or ended Evan's treatment before it had begun.

When beginning treatments, I stress to parents not only that they have the right and privilege to call me on anything that strikes them as wrong, ill-advised, tactless, worrisome, threatening, or slighting but that they have an obligation to do so. I explain that without honesty, a relationship has little else. Frustration, hurt, or anger that goes underground, I further explain, doesn't disappear or resolve on its own but is more likely to fester under the surface, where it can impede our work and the child's therapy.

It's a rare week when I don't have one or two parents question something I say or do, mini-confrontations that get easier for parents to carry out and that almost always strengthen our connection and mutual trust. My inviting demand also counters some of what by nature can be an imbalanced relationship between the (authoritative and powerful) therapist and the (helpless and help-seeking) parents. After all, the child therapist routinely questions parents. Why shouldn't they have the same right and duty in return?

When treating a child from a two-parent family, whether intact or divorced, we often find it's one parent who "does" the therapy thing for the family, one parent who makes the appointments, transports the child, and comes to parent meetings. What do child therapists make of and do about this situation? With many children, the mother brings the children to therapy no differently than she does the doctor's visits, soccer practice, and the rest. But I need to wonder when I find that one parent assumes responsibility for the therapy business even though she works her own job as much or more than the father I seldom see. I may find a simple answer, as when a one-parent show reflects a family's divisions of labor—one parent does the gymnastics, one parent does music lessons, and one parent does therapy. In other families the lopsided arrangement is more telling; it is the more willing and motivated parent who brings the child to our offices and clinics.

Although we allow ourselves to observe and imagine all that we want and parents' underlying motives are relevant to what we do and how we'll do it, our main interest is not in analyzing their unconscious. Our mission is to engage both parents in the child's treatment. Merely inviting the second parent may suffice. Once we've met and connected with the other parent, we may start seeing more of him or her around the waiting room or on the telephone. Rather than insist on their presence, I tend to ask for it. I stress how their input might assist me. "It'd really help my work with James if I could get *your* thoughts and observations." As is true for most of us, parents like knowing that what they think and feel is significant, particularly when feeling the vulnerability of having sought and needed an outside expert's help.

I use the same approach with parents who don't live in the same house or when their availability in the child's life is limited. Bad reputations generally don't dissuade me from trying. I strive to remain open and neutral to hearing everyone's side of the parenting story. Parents on the outs, as are many divorced fathers, can surprise us with their love, concerns, and insights into the child. Fathers whom I persuade to come in by themselves express surprise that I bother and care to hear from them. I have seen these men profoundly moved that the therapist has acknowledged their place and influence in their child's world.

How and why did they get estranged from their child's life, my questioning will aim to discover. Although these parents usually first talk with blame and anger of how they were pushed out, they soon after may confess ways in which they themselves detached, pulled away, or abdicated all their parental authority and caretaking to their spouse. True, as you're thinking, the in-the-home and in-the-therapy spouse is not always overjoyed to have their ex back in the picture. But it's usually good for the therapy and the child and, in the long run, the at-home parent too.

What do we do when a spouse will have nothing to do with us or the therapy? I've met many mothers who, even with my assistance, can't get their husbands to come in. Frequently, we have to go forward without his presence and input. Some few mothers have used me to help bring the therapy and parenting guidance home to their husband or significant other. Instead of their using his absence or what I say as a weapon against him, these mothers fairly and compassionately have represented him in the process, expressing *his* worries and complaints and problem solving constructive ways to support his own growth as a parent at home. This superhuman dynamic is a marvel to watch and admire and appears to be more than most parents, men or women, can do.

I must be careful, however, not to leave the impression that I or any other child therapist can make therapeutic contact with any and every parent.

> The divorced and estranged father of a boy I saw stood out on the sidewalk. "I'm not coming in there," he announced loudly, seeming not to care who heard him. He held his hand up for me to not come nearer. "We can talk from there," he said as he backed into the road. "I don't know why you called me, but I changed my mind. I think it's better if we don't meet."
>
> "I thought you might be able to help me understand Ty," I said. I knew this man was unreliable, unpredictable, and occasionally violent. But even if he had been to prison and had a heroin problem, he was my patient's father. "If you'd like, we can talk out here."
>
> "It's okay, thanks," Ty's father said, looking a lot like a cornered animal. He jumped in his car and sped off. I tried calling once more, but he never called back.

Sadly, there are too many parents who can't or won't parent and who can't or won't participate in their child's therapy. Their problems are often varied and multiple: alcohol, drugs, crime, violence, irresponsibility, and immaturity, to name a few. What do we do with the children? We try to counter and undo such children's common belief that they are the problem, that they must be unlovable and undeserving of good love and caring. We strive to help them shed their hurts and to realize that the problem lies in their parents' incapacity to love and care. And while we promote the children's growing more willing and able to protect and stand up for themselves, to find good love and caring from good people, we support their wishes, when they arise, to forgive those who've mistreated or neglected them.

According to the Peace Corps model, it is more empowering to teach people to grow their own food than it is to feed them. Likewise, even more than giving mothers and fathers our concrete and practical suggestions, we aim to broaden, deepen, sensitize, and enlighten their parenting. Foremost, we want to help parents better see and recognize their children's needs, for sensing needs is requisite to filling them.

"I called your coach today," Wen's mother said, as she handed him a small brown lunch bag. "He said it's okay if you miss the game Friday to go to Gretchen's birthday party." Wen, a 12-year-old boy with depression, gave his mother an exasperated nod, then looked at me. "See what I mean," he said.

"But you told me you wanted to go to Gretchen's party."

"Her party is Saturday morning at the trampoline place."

"Who has a party Saturday morning? That's kind of weird, don't you think?" his mother asked me.

Wen had told me many times about how his mother never seemed to get it right. She made a lot of noise and commotion about doing for him. "She likes to think she's a great mother," he explained with his typical acuity.

Wen reached into the bag. He took out and opened a sandwich wrapped in foil. Again, frustration.

"What's the matter? I made it on white bread like you asked."

Wen sighed. "I said they told us that oatmeal and rye breads are healthier."

"I thought you don't like breads that are heavier and grainy?"

"That's *what you said*."

Readers who haven't heard all that I had might wonder if Wen wasn't a bit spoiled and critical of his mother. But—and you'll have to take my word on it—he was actually a pretty kindly and patient boy. With an uncanny sense, as if she didn't really want to satisfy him, Wen's mother constantly made efforts on his behalf that somehow missed the mark. She'd stop on her way home from work to buy him her favorite flavor ice cream. She'd observe that he looked tired when she'd stayed up too late and would ask about his English quiz the night after he'd studied for a math test.

"So, if I have it right," I said. "Your mother wants to do nice things for you. But it just never feels right."

"Not never," Wen corrected me, willing to give an inch in exchange for the confirming I'd given him. "I know she loves me. It just seems like she doesn't listen or care what I tell her."

Wen watched his mother closely. He didn't miss her reddening eyes. "How'd your personnel review meeting go today?" he asked.

"Good," his mother nodded, smiling through her tears. "Good." She looked to me. "He always remembers what I tell him."

Wen walked to his mother and put his arm around her.

"Who's taking care of who?" she asked me, her head resting on her 12-year-old's shoulder.

It'd taken a fair number of meetings for Wen's mother to get to this place. Recognizing one's own self-absorption is a tough admission. The issue glared at us the first time we'd met, and yet what good would it have done for me to have then pointed out how she confused Wen's needs with her own? I would have succeeded in making her feel like a worse mother than she already judged herself to be. We might wish that hearing such a truth would shock a parent to climb out of herself and be more responsive to her child. But people who are parents don't work that neatly, especially those consumed by their own perspective and needs. Our assaulting their self-esteem makes them hurt more and opens wounds, in turn making them more fragile and needing to feed, soothe, and steady themselves above and before all others.

The unrelenting press of her own needs sometimes blinded Wen's mother to those of her son's. But other parents withhold their responsiveness more deliberately, out of hurt or anger. It is hard to give empathy and caring to someone who you believe dislikes you. Many parents feel rejected and unloved by their own child, a child who's intentionally mean to them or one whose personality they mistake for personal affront. Breaking these vicious cycles—child reacts to parent reacts to child reacts to parent reacts to. . .—takes therapists' steady and patient work over time. As the "bad" child grows nicer and even remorseful, parents can rediscover the love and empathy they once knew, just as parents of the different child may come to accept his ways as who he is rather than as willful rejection of their affection and themselves.

Just as we work to help parents see children's needs more clearly, we work to help them perceive their children more realistically. Parent guidance can effectively help parents to recognize their children's real interests, abilities, and liabilities. For every parent who wants her severely learning disabled daughter to go to Yale, there's one who doesn't expect enough of her. Some parents coddle their physically handicapped children; others race them down ski slopes. Child therapists can help tease out parents' fears and disappointment, clearing out the way so they can hold renewed and realistic hope for what a child might accomplish, just as it can temper excessive expectations in a parent who has yet to come to terms with and grieve a child's disability or illness. Rigid and two-dimensional assumptions, whether underestimating or overreaching, misread the complexity and richness of real children and leave them stuck in bad places. Our therapies implicitly and explicitly remind the parents we work with that each of us has limitations. It's how children learn to accept, cope with, and overcome their limitations that will determine how well they adapt and how far they progress.

Parent guidance is a useful term to describe our meetings. And yet, those meetings often take turns or evolve into something more. Helping a parent figure out better strategies for discipline sounds like guidance. But what do we call our listening to a sobbing father who, in dealing with his own absence from the home and the children, recalls his own abusive and neglecting dad? What do we call a mother who spends her hour spewing her anger at the way her ex-husband dotes more on his new stepchildren? And what do we call it when a mother and father bicker, attack, or sit coldly and silently at opposite ends of the office?

Skilled and effective supervisors of therapy learn how to help trainees balance their issues with those of the patients. For a supervisor to over-indulge therapists'-in-training own stuff makes it more like their therapy and abandons the clinical work and the patient. But to exclude trainees' feelings, issues, and tears from supervision comparably risks making the supervision narrow, superficial, and impotent. In a parallel universe, child therapists invite and listen to any emotional expression, revelation, or insight that can help a mother or father to better see and parent their child.

How powerfully informative it can be for me to sit uncomfortably between warring parents. I can tell them firsthand how awful it feels for me, a well-trained and analyzed grown-up, to be helplessly caught between them. Better yet, I can ask them what they imagine their hour of fighting has been like for me. Their answer will spontaneously go to the child they love. Their willingness to bring me their troubled marriage allows me to understand and talk of how their competitiveness, resentment, or hatred for one another clouds and contaminates their parenting decisions and behavior. It also will bring to the fore their guilt and pain over the way their endless battle hurts their child.

When facing parents whose own issues or poor marriages seem to loom larger than what parent guidance can do, we may gently wonder aloud whether they might wish more help in that area—for example, a marriage counselor or an individual therapist. When doing so, we take great care to not make the parent feel rejected or bad for having brought their hurts to us. Nor do we wish to give the wrong message, that they should keep themselves out of our meetings. Nothing could be farther from the truth. In the end, it is the therapist's responsibility, not theirs, to put whatever parents bring in to good therapeutic use for the sake of the child. In my experience as a clinician and supervisor, this is one of the most difficult and critical aspects of the child therapist's work.

In this regard, I wish to make special mention of our work with single mothers. As I cowrote elsewhere, "millions of single mothers trek miles each day" carrying babies on their backs and groceries and diaper bags in their arms, never getting enough sleep and yet still cooking and cleaning and, often, working, even when sick. Many single-mother families live in poverty or have far less than they and their families need; many receive little sympathy and compassion. These dedicated parents push themselves beyond limits—not for a weeklong expedition but for months and years on end—out of concern for their child's well-being, demonstrating every day of their lives the real stuff of human spirit and purpose. All too often, a single mother has to clear an unrealistically high hurdle, be an Erin Brockovich or mother of a U.S. president to win our notice and approval. Who are the real heroes?" (Bromfield and Erwin, 2001, p. 291). Any one who has been a parent in an intact marriage can only wonder how a single mother does it alone. And the statistics make her job yet more daunting. Children of single mothers are at greater peril of academic failure, delinquency, substance abuse, criminal behavior, depression, failed marriages, on and on.

It's easy to see why I am highly motivated to do everything I can to help support a single mother's parenting. I teach, encourage, listen, cajole, whatever. If a single mother needs to use me as a therapist today, I oblige. I know that the last thing she can afford is another hour out of her crazy schedule. Knowing that she lacks the money or time or maybe the initiative to get to the bookstore, I will not hesitate to give her a book that I think might benefit her and her child. If she tells me about a bad business idea or getting ripped off by an auto garage, I may help her find the number for the consumer hotline or reputable car mechanic. Fostering social supports, obtaining physical help, and learning to nurture themselves become centerpieces of our work with single mothers. In addition to the obvious assistance our helping hands can give, they also symbolically tell a single mother that the trials of her daily life are seen and appreciated, that her efforts to parent well are noted and worthy.

Hardly last—two meager chapters cannot do justice to the world of parent guidance—I wish to mention the occasional request we get to meet with people who are contemplating adoption. When parents ask if I might help them think through their decision, I feel compelled to do whatever I can to provide them an honest and open space to do so. Why? Working with many adopted children and families has taught me what a responsibility it can be. Whether in using me as a sounding board or by reading books that I recommend (e.g., Varon, 2000), parents coming to clearer terms with what adopting means to them can only be good. It's far better to realize now, instead of years into a childhood, that one really doesn't have the resources, commitment, and energy to raise a child. And, for the majority of prospective parents who do go on to adopt, they take surer steps on a foundation of foresight, information, and preparation.

When it comes to the parent work of child therapy, I envision our role something like the hockey goalie who does anything and everything—standing tall; sprawling sideways; stopping pucks with his glove, his stick, and his pads; saving goals with grace and with clumsier moves; watching plays evolve from the other end of the ice or catching a flash of rubber in a split second; combining years of playing with reflex; study of the game with what he feels in his gut; and using every last ounce of who he is to do his job. As child therapists, we need to use it all—our experience, training, technique, intuition, smarts, reason, conscience, empathy, and so on—to try our best to forge meaningful connections with the parents who our child patients love and need. Whatever we think of the parents, our purpose is to support their doing better by their children. To do anything less, make no mistake, lets down and fails the child, undermining the very therapy we work so hard to establish and carry on.

13

On Brotherly Love and Musical Chairs: Family Work

Children mostly live in families, and that has everything to do with their circumstances and who they are. Even clinicians who do individual child therapy may spend considerable time and attention thinking about and working with other members of the child's family. In this chapter we will talk more about meetings between parents and children as well as those that involve siblings.

Given what can go on in my waiting room, it's a wonder I don't invite a parent into every one of the child's hours.

"'Cause you're an asshole. That's why." The door to my office was partly opened.

"I don't see what the big thing is," his mother replied. "I would have been happy to do it myself. But I thought you'd have wanted to introduce me to your coach."

"Yeah, well you thought wrong."

"I still don't get why—"

"I told you."

"I didn't hear it."

"'Cause . . . you . . . are . . .," Martin spoke slowly and clearly. "A . . . big . . . asshole."

Although my door was open, I knocked on it before going out to the waiting room. Who could be sure? Maybe Martin hadn't known I could hear everything.

"Martin's mad at me," his mother began. "I thought he might introduce me—"

"You're an asshole. You're an asshole." Martin's words, if calm and rhythmic, were enough to block his mother's words. "You're an asshole." Martin got up, gave his mother the finger, and walked into the office.

"Why don't you come in, too?" I invited, gesturing to his mother.

"Okay, but he won't like that," she replied, looking here-goes-nothing.

"You're an asshole," Martin said once more as his mother took a seat, confirming any doubt as to who his performance was for.

Martin grinned. Although constantly angry and frustrated, he seldom could articulate what was upsetting him. It instead would come out in a chronic and tiring stream of sarcasm, put downs, and oppositional behavior. I didn't ask him what bothered him because I'd asked that many times previously. He hated that question and would respond with a curt "nothing" and withdraw. I stood a better chance of engaging a cursing Martin than one giving me the cold shoulder.

And Martin's cold shoulder was frigid. For our first dozen or so meetings, he'd sat with his back to me reading the thick adult thrillers he adored. A passing observer—or even a researcher on the efficacy of psychotherapy—might have judged our meetings to be a waste. What could possibly be therapeutic about a therapist silently watching a child read? They wouldn't have sensed the deep satisfaction Martin felt in his shunning of me. Nor would they have stayed long enough to see him linger at the hour's end. They surely wouldn't have heard the parents and school staff report that his bullying and disrupting had markedly lessened. Martin was obviously getting something out of this safe opportunity to give an important person in his life (which I represented) a hard time. But he had miles of growth to go. He was often irritable and aggressive with his mother, so much so that she had moments when she feared him.

"Why does he think you're such an asshole?" I asked.

"'Cause she just is," Martin spoke out. I turned to his mother. She faltered. Martin jumped in again. "'Cause she's an asshole."

I might have "thrown" Martin out of the office, but to what end? I might have tried to exercise some authority, telling him that his language wasn't acceptable (but he knew I didn't feel that way). Not to mention, his father and teachers, who were bigger than I, had given him plenty of tough love with little results.

"Maybe he just doesn't want me to hear what you're going to say," I said casually. "But I do, so go ahead. Please."

In her usual rambling way, Martin's mother went on to describe how she'd taken him to soccer, how she hadn't had a problem with sports because she thought they were good for him, how she'd known the coach's sister several years ago . . .

Martin screamed. "Shut up! This is what I can't stand." He stood up and began to fling dominoes at the wall. With each bullet, his might and anger rose. He eyed daggers at his mother as he shouted. "I hate the way you talk." "I hate the way you take forever to say anything." "I hate the way you get sick."

Martin's eyes watered. "Fuck you! Fuck this." He whipped the basket of dominoes at the wall and fell into his chair. He covered his face with his arm. I gestured for Martin's mother to leave. She tiptoed out and shut the door behind her.

"She gets sick?" I asked Martin quietly.

"All the time," he said with tears. "She's been sick my whole fucking life."

When Martin was a toddler, his mother had taken to bed for an unknown illness. Since then, he described, she'd spent a lot of time in bed, that is, when she wasn't going off to yoga retreats, meditating, or shushing his laughter because she had a migraine. "And you hate her for being sick?" I asked. "I hate her for making me feel like I made her sick," he shot back. That one meeting between mother and son hardly resolved everything. We had many such meetings, and each brought a dollop of peace to their relationship.

Why had I invited her in to Martin's hour? I knew their relation-ship was terribly conflicted. Their skirmish in my waiting room had handed me a silver-plated opportunity to address it firsthand. Why had I allowed Martin to talk so fresh to his mother? I don't think that I could have stopped it. Even had I been able to, I'd have only gotten him to play nice in the office, leaving them to go home as miserable as they'd come. And why had I permitted him to throw dominoes at my wall? That, in my opinion, beat his pushing a classmate through a glass door or verbally abusing his mother. I feared that Martin would become physically aggressive with his mother and eventually with his future girlfriends or wife.

Beside parents and children who argue, what else do child therapists find in their waiting rooms? Coddling parents who'll do anything to entertain their children, asking perhaps if the four-course snack they brought is okay? Estranged families sitting as far from each other as they can. Disorganized families moving the furniture, switching the radio station, and making messes. Powerless parents watching helplessly as their children play with light switches or open cookie boxes despite five warnings to the contrary. Neglecting parents, too busy with their cell phones or laptops to notice when their child needs a tissue or wanders off. Inevitably, children and their parents bring their real-world issues to our waiting rooms, and, sometimes, child therapists can put that to good use by inviting everyone in.

Rather than last minute, child therapists can also plan a meeting to bring parent and child together. I often do this in an attempt to avert what appears to be a brewing crisis, as I did with Antonio, a high school junior who was heading full speed toward a crash with his parents. In his weekly hour, Antonio complained that his parents were overly strict and demanding. In their parent guidance sessions, his parents complained that Antonio was lazy and irresponsible. I brought them together expect-ing an explosive blame game. I witnessed exactly the opposite, a group confessional that led to more considerate behavior on everyone's part.

The reasons that child therapists arrange such meetings vary and can include the goals of facilitating better communication, defusing anger that is mounting or at a loggerhead, enhancing relationships, and modi-fying dysfunctional behaviors. Child and teen patients have requested that I ask a parents in so that they, with my support, can express some-thing difficult over which they fear repercussions. Parents and children have asked to meet with the other because they "can't live like this any-more." I've frequently offered joint parent–child sessions to spotlight a developmental phase, as I did with Catie, a 15-year-old girl with Down syndrome.

Catie was a jewel. The daughter of two college professors, she was what I conceptualize to be gifted within the context of her disability. She loved school and her teachers. She loved romantic movies and danc-ing. She loved her classmates and friends. She loved her mother and her father and her sister and brother-in-law—*dearly*. She loved everyone, so she said. Unfortunately, she'd show this love indiscriminately, hugging people she hardly knew or holding too long and too hard on to those she did know. This behavior annoyed her family, tested her teachers' patience, and, so we feared, made her vulnerable with strangers. And yet, I didn't want to simply use behavioral techniques to extinguish her hugs as undesirable behavior. They held too much meaning for such a shallow and potentially cruel intervention.

The answer didn't crystallize until quite some time later in Catie's treatment. She'd come to her session uncharacteristically angry, cursing about a girl "who stole her man." As she told me her story, it appeared to me that this girl had done Catie wrong. Fortified by my listening and support, Catie had decided to confront the girl the next day by asking her a carefully scripted and rehearsed question. "How could you kiss my boyfriend? I thought we were best friends." Catie left the office with a bounce in her step, feeling, she said, like a strong and independent woman who would speak her mind.

When I went out to greet Catie the next week, I expected to find a glowing and confident girl. Catie avoided my eyes. She walked somberly to my office with her eyes to the floor. She sat stiffly in her chair and brought up many subjects, all mundane and going nowhere. She said nothing about her friend. Finally, I asked her why she wasn't looking at me. "I'm sorry," she blurted. "I let you down. I couldn't do it. I can't be a bitch."

Over the next many months, Catie talked in detail about her fear of hurting people and making them mad. "If I yell at them," she said, "they won't love me anymore." With much pain, Catie compiled lists of insults and injuries she'd suffered the day and week before. She started off with trivial slights, such as someone not holding the door. She even-tually spoke of being mocked at a dance and of being treated differently because she had Down syndrome. This work came to a head after a weekend during which her mother had gone away. Catie and her father had planned a "date" to go to her favorite restaurant for dinner and then come home to watch Audrey Hepburn in *Breakfast at Tiffany's*. But her usually attentive father had forgotten. He'd arranged for a friend to come over to watch baseball and eat pizza. Catie took a TV dinner to her room and watched the movie by herself.

"He cheated on me," Catie lamented.

"You were so disappointed," I said. "You were counting on him."

Catie forcibly held her tears in check. Her face reddened. "I am so fucking pissed off," she said, using a curse I'd never heard her say. "Who does he think he is? I've got a life too. I'm not no nobody!" Catie stood up, pushed her chair to the ground, and marched toward the door.

"Where are you going?"

"That's my business!" Catie tugged the door open and stomped toward the waiting room.

With glee, I peeked down the hall. Hearing her confront her father was going to be music to my ears. But I heard something else. "I love you, Daddy. You're the best Daddy in the whole world." She hugged her father and wouldn't let go, so much in fact, that her father, with Catie glued on, walked to my office and asked if he might come in.

"She does this all the time." Catie's father tactfully tried to slip his daughter's arms off his neck.

"That's because I love you so much," Catie said in a saccharine and whiny voice.

"I know you love me, and I love you," her father replied. Each time he undid her arms, they reattached, as if tentacles. "But it doesn't always feel good."

"Catie," I said. "Would you like me to tell your father what you're really feeling?"

Catie let go of her father, moved her chair next to mine, and sat down.

"I know it looks like Catie is feeling all love," I began. "But she's feeling something else right now." I began to tell her story, but Catie cut me off. She told him everything, except, instead of telling him off, she told him why she couldn't tell him off.

Feeling understood, Catie's response surprised both her father and myself. "I know my hugs go over the top," she said. "But I don't know how to hug right when I'm so mad at somebody. Are you mad at me?" she asked her father.

"Of course not." He opened up his arms for a warm hug that was not at all clingy.

Following that session, Catie and I worked on ways to hug, hand-shake, and high five. Ways to say hello and say good-bye. Ways to meet new people and ways to love dear friends and family. We also talked of ways to let people know what she really felt without having to worry that she'd lose their love or respect.

Family meetings can serve as a good forum to discuss important life decisions. Tray was a good athlete but a horrible student. He barely made it through his first year of college and dreaded returning for his sophomore year. His parents feared that if he quit school he'd never return. We held a series of joint meetings to figure this out. I made clear in the first few minutes that we were in no rush and that we'd take as long, as many sessions, as it took us to come to a comfortable and sound conclusion. Problem solving is a process, I stressed, and has to run its course. And so we spent an initial hour lamenting how bad the previous year had been. Tray's parents vented their frustrations while speaking too of their belief that their son needed to go back and fin-ish college. Tray admitted that he didn't care about school and that he felt he was wasting his parents' hard-earned money. Everyone left this first session looking defeated, hopeless, and confused. In the second hour, however, the parents were coming to believe that their son must grow up according to his own developmental timetable. They heard his argument to go work for a year and learn to live more on his own. His plan to pursue community college, a plan they'd earlier balked at, was starting to sound to them less like failure and more like a hopeful, realistic, and responsible choice. By the end of the third meeting, the parents happily endorsed their son's decision to withdraw from school and to begin building his life on a more personal and slower timetable. Several years later, after this young man graduated from a state college with good grades and many accomplishments, both he and his family had come to see that moment of crisis as the turning point toward his maturation and success.

Parents can employ these family meetings and my help when establishing new rules for the household. Using the therapy room for a family
council offers advantages to their doing it at home. The office is a safe
place where a family can rely on me to keep things in control and constructive. Some parents feel my presence can help to ensure their child's
listening to and hearing their messages. I allow the space and time for
everyone to express their feelings, which itself can enable all parties to
come to a well-defined agreement. I've seen more than a few parents call
for late summer and early fall pow-wows to set the stage for the upcoming academic year or transition to a new school. It's not unusual for me
to mediate parent–child discussions on relevant topics such as bedtime,
homework, use of computers, and the like. These meetings work so well
that, once experienced, families put them in their toolbox of parenting
tools for later use. Perhaps, more than anything and for all of the humor
we commonly share, our holding a group meeting can add a gravity and
purpose that moves both parent and child to take their negotiations
more seriously and to heart.

There are no concrete guidelines for conducting parent–child meetings. They can be short or long, single shots or repeated over time,
urgent or planned. I treat teens whose parents I rarely see and children
whose parents pop in and out of every session. There are situations in
which I work to keep parents out of the office, and there are others
where they are ever welcome, especially at the child's behest. It all comes
down to what works for a particular treatment and family. Therapists
can train parents to expect and utilize such sessions. It's a skill that both
therapist and parents can acquire.

Second in frequency to parent–child meetings are those that involve
siblings. Many of the children who come for therapy have complicated
relationships with their bothers and sisters. Signs of that conflict can
be overt jealousies and aggression directly aimed at a sibling as well as
disguised envy and excessive competition that shows itself in the classroom or on the playground. In some families, friction between siblings
can be mollified in a session or two, as it did for two sisters who fought
endlessly.

My patient, eight-year-old Lana, comfortably drew at my desk with
her back to Lauren, her 11-year-old sister, who sat nervously across
from me.

"So, you say, Lana embarrasses you?" I repeated to Lauren.

"She tags along everywhere and acts really immature."

"That's 'cause you had your friend, Maggie, but Susie was sick," Lana piped in without looking up from her crayons and paper.

"Anyway," Lauren continued as if brushing a fly off her leg, "Lauren attacks me like some kind of animal. She scratches and bites me."

"I only bit you once, and that's 'cause you were holding my hands." Lauren raised her eyebrows as if to say, See what I mean?

I'd been seeing Lana for many months. She'd been referred for her impulsivity, short fuse, moodiness, and aggressiveness. I knew she could be a tough and pestering sister. She'd told me herself. But we'd made considerable gains on all fronts, and that was what had made this meeting of sisters a possibility and what had led to Lana's explicitly asking for it.

"And she's like disgusting," Lauren added. "She picks her nose and eats it."

"I do not eat it!" Lana interrupted, this accusation, true or not, being the last straw. Lana turned to face me. "She hates me," she said. "She's always hated me. I can't stand it." If I'd been a parent, Lana would have run to my arms for reassurance. She stood by my chair and confronted Lauren. "Why don't you like me? I love *you*!"

"I don't hate you," Lauren said. "You're just a bothersome little sister."

"You do hate me," Lana screamed back through tears. "I heard you tell Mom that you wished I was dead."

Lauren blushed and herself started to cry, mostly out of shame that she really had spoken those words. "But I, I, I didn't mean it," she stuttered.

Lana leaned against my shoulder, sobbing deeply. "But you said it."

The hour ended pretty much there—Lana seemingly in despair and her older sister humiliated and guilt-ridden. "Good work, girls," I said, smiling at them as I handed them both tissues to take for the road. I got a call that night from their mother who reported that the girls had planned and cooked the family dinner that night and that they'd had the most fun she'd seen her daughters have in ages. As my treatment of Lana proceeded, we occasionally invited Lauren in, and it always brought a measure of relief and resolution to both girls. In many other families, sadly, the animosity between siblings is too great for a children-only meeting. Consider Justin, a very troubled teen whose hatred for his younger brother approached homicidal proportions.

Justin's parents had brought him to me out of fear that he might irrevocably harm Kendall. Justin would forever bump and poke Kendall, giving him unwanted wedgies, head noogies, and knuckles in his thighs. Justin would get Kendall in headlocks and not let him go. There was ample name-calling too, calling his younger brother "homo," "retard," and the rest. When Justin barely missed his brother's eye with a field hockey stick, his parents realized they couldn't put treatment off any longer.

When we met as a family, I could easily understand Justin's jealousy. Kendall was cute, funny, bright, congenial, articulate, emotionally expressive, socially at ease, everything Justin wasn't. Justin was odd looking, self-conscious, awkward, obsessive, and overflowing with anger. Throughout this first meeting, everything that Kendall said or did infuriated Justin, who dedicated his part of the hour to ridiculing, mimicking, and generally trying to discredit his brother. Oh, and as you can guess, Kendall got along with his parents well; Justin did not. It would have been easy to put two and two together in that initial meeting. If I had, though, I would have come up with the wrong answer.

It wasn't until the third or fourth parent meeting that the calculus of this family started to tease out. Justin's parents had stormed in ahead of the boys, furious that he'd ruined the family's Thanksgiving dinner.

"He attacked Kendall?" I asked.

"He literally jumped across the table and grabbed his collar," his father described, holding his own shirt to demonstrate. "Justin actually pulled him across the table."

"Justin doesn't realize how much bigger and stronger he is," his mother added.

"He dragged me through the mash potatoes and squash," Kendall quipped while nonchalantly toying with a Hacky Sack and seeming to enjoy the drama. Justin stared ahead, his fists clenched.

"It makes no sense," his father said. "Absolutely no provocation. A blatant attack."

Just at that moment, I noticed Kendall mouth something to his brother. Justin went after Kendall, but I stepped in between. "Hold on," I urged.

At that juncture, I had everyone's attention. Justin's parents wanted to know what was happening. Kendall was fearing what I might say. And Justin hoped for some desperately needed vindication.

"What were you saying?" I asked Kendall. He squirmed and sidled to his mother, where he hid his face behind her shoulder. His mother gently but firmly nudged him back into view. No one spoke. We waited. After several tense minutes, Kendall broke down.

"I was just having fun." He was crying out of fear, but no one seemed to feel much sympathy.

"What did you say?" the boys' father asked sternly. Kendall ran behind a chair and yelled the word, "Booberry!"

Justin chuckled, and we all laughed.

"Booberry?" I repeated to be sure.

"Booberry," Justin confirmed.

Justin explained how, a couple of years earlier, his brother had told him that everyone loved him better than Justin. He'd point out how much handsomer, funnier, happier, and easier he was to be with. Kendall loved to egg Justin to lose his temper and go after him, for those were the times when his parents would swoop in like eagles to rescue and coddle him. "Booberry," a babyish version of blueberry, had become the silent and secret code that represented everything about that painful and sorry dynamic. The jig was up, the mystery unraveled. "And to think it was Justin who really needed our protection all this time," his mother concluded.

Meetings between siblings are not limited to rivalry and in-fighting. Brothers and sisters have effectively used me and the office to work out feelings related to a sibling's special needs, to a sibling going off to college, and to a sibling having been mistreated by the other. I've held meetings where an older sibling has come in out of concern for a younger one's troubles and where step- and half-siblings have met to turn themselves into family. I've met, too, with siblings who come together not because they fight but to support each other as they both or all cope with family tragedy, illness, and divorce.

There's no end to the configurations and aims of the family work that child therapists inevitably employ. Whether meeting with parents and children, siblings, grandparents, nannies, or other caretakers, we strive to creatively bring together whoever is part of the problem and solution,

ever in the service of making the child's and family's life less burdened
and more harmonious. The child therapist who is open to and skilled in
working with families cannot help but be a more effective and satisfied
clinician.[1]

NOTE

1. I am not a family therapist. I have neither the training nor the skills for
it. As you have read, my family work is organized around a therapy with an
individual child. Some family therapists, I understand, do not see individuals
as much as they see a family system. I do not have that kind of vision. When
families call me looking for or in need of true family therapy, I refer them
on. This is a long way of saying that I am not recommending resources in
family therapy, for readers will likely better know where to look and who
to ask. For that matter, a majority of readers could probably advise me on
this matter.

14

Talking Heads: Working with Schools and Other Agencies

On the average, children in therapy spend about six days and 23 hours without us. Although we meet with the child for only an hour or so, we therapists often become the child's unofficial liaison to the rest of her life, a life that can largely take place in a school. As the child's therapist, we have something to offer teachers and school staff to better understand and help her. As the child's therapist, we also have much to learn from them, information and feedback that can help us to better understand and work with our patient. This chapter addresses the child therapist's role as consultant to schools and other agencies, such as courts and social services.

What, we need to know at the outset, do we wish to accomplish? Why do we want to make contact with a child's school? We pursue obvious goals, like garnering information as to how the child is faring academically, socially, and so on. We might wish to know what services a child receives, how frequently, and by what personnel. And we want to give teachers information in return, sharing what we can to help them in their work with the child. These, however, are mere generalities of a child therapist's work with schools. Let's examine some details and examples of this critical, frequent, often complex, and challenging aspect of being a child therapist.

Before I describe how I conceptualize school consultation—consultation meaning communication specifically related to one of my child patients—we should discuss the more traditional approach. In my experience, clinicians and teachers most commonly come together for occasional and formal team meetings as part of individualized (special) education plans. We all know these meetings, where teachers, guidance, administrators, and outside clinicians share input and problem solve as a group. What happens at these meetings? Many things—some good, some not so good, and lots of group dynamics, much of it diverting. At their best, a team of professionals contribute keen insights that cohere into a well-meaning and well-informed discussion that, in turn, leads to doable and smart decisions on behalf of the child's immediate and distant future. At their worst, they turn into pig piles of complaining about difficult children who disrupt, annoy, bother, and ruin everyone's day. Of course, a majority of team meetings fall somewhere between these two extremes.

Some of what endows these meetings with structure and due process is also what can curtail their effectiveness as a place and time for the therapist's optimal consulting. There is often an enormous or pressing agenda that needs to get done in short order. Listening is sort of a leisurely endeavor and one that is often crowded out of the room by too much to do in too little time by people who have other fires burning, tests to correct, lessons to plan. The meetings are routinely run by administrators who have to get something accomplished, settled, and agreed on. The goal probably sounds more like what are we going to do with Billy (i.e., what classroom, what placement, what medicine) than how can we raise our mutual awareness of Billy's experiences as he goes through his school day.

At some point in the meeting, the child's therapist will be asked to speak his mind. Child psychotherapists, being attuned to and interested in what a child experiences, have a tendency to go on about that sort of thing, perhaps getting back funny looks and circumspect comments that basically ask, "Can you just get real, get practical, get with the program?"

Does the skill for communicating in a group setting correspond to the skill of doing therapy? Probably not, though they are both valuable, for sure.

Child therapists are in a vulnerable position. They, of course, can blow in—as some of us are apt to do—as the self-important authorities who's going to tell everyone how it is and should be. Such arrogance seldom generates good feeling for therapists and fosters a resentment that will rub off (and may unconsciously be taken out) on the child, especially a child who himself can be selfish, demanding, and all that. On the other hand, child therapists have to rise above the groupthink that can dominate meetings. They must resist the pressure to just agree or say what will please others or avoid an issue lest it cause trouble, extra work, or impossible demands for other professionals at the meeting.

Conflict of interest can be a reckoning force at such meetings. Some child therapists, who for all of their lofty goals still must pay the rent and college tuitions, may not feel wholly free to say or do what they believe is best for the child. Many child therapists find themselves burning the candle at both ends, wanting to keep the patient and his family happy while also wanting to get along with school personnel who have potential patients to refer. Schools tend to refer children and families to the therapists they know and can count on to work with them, which means who won't make waves or ask for too much. The child therapist who gets too cozy with a school, consciously or unawares, may need to compromise his efforts on behalf of any one child. This can result in weakened educational planning, avoidance of responsibility and difficult conversations, and insincere double-talk (i.e., bad-mouthing the family to the school while bad-mouthing the school to the parent). That so much can be at stake in what may be once-a-year meetings only accentuates the problem.

Some therapists, on the other hand, are facile at these meetings. They comfortably commute between the child and the goal, between inner experience and outer reality, between what a therapist does and what a teacher and a school can do. These therapists can ferret out the underlying agenda from that on the surface, placing the child's needs square center on the table. They are able to frame the child's perspective in language that is accessible and clear to nonclinicians, translating complex and subtle experiences into concepts that make sense and bear relevance to the classroom. They come to meetings prepared, having envisioned what the child would receive in an ideal world, then downsizing that impossibility to an optimized version of what would be ideal in the world of that particular and real school. By fostering strong, trusting, and communicative relationships with school personnel, such therapists establish a solid position to help schools help their patients. Few child therapists can do all this at once and well. We try our best to do as much of it as we can, learning from each meeting what we can to do it better next time.

As readers have probably started to sense, over the years I have developed a somewhat different approach to my work with schools. Rather than use the team meeting, I much prefer to develop an ongoing relationship with one or two persons at the school, preferably a person who is reliable, has good feeling for the child, and is open to reflection about the case and whom the parents hold some trust in. But that is a wish list. I always try to establish a connection with the person who lives in the trenches with the child, the teacher. In situations when the teacher doesn't like the child, I strive to see her perspective and grasp why she might not want an outsider's input. If I want to win her over to the child's perspective, I try hard to show that I get hers.

How do I begin to establish a relationship with a child's teacher? I approach her (or him) with consideration for her own being. I e-mail or call, leaving a brief message that identifies myself as the child's therapist and that says I'd very much appreciate hearing her insights as to how the child is doing and that asks if we might speak at some time that is convenient for her. No rush, I always add. When we finally connect, I ask again to make sure. "Is this a good time?" People make demands on teachers all day long.

While I introduce myself as the child's therapist, I make clear that I call not to give my opinion but to hear hers. I ask open-ended questions that invite her candid and usually insightful observations. "How's it looking?" I might ask. "He must be a handful." "What's your sense of how the year is going?" I listen and don't interrupt. I don't argue, critique, or rush to prove her wrong. After all, as his teacher, she spends long days after days with our patient. I may disagree with her interpretations of what his behaviors signify, but that doesn't diminish her authority as an educator who knows him well. Teachers always have much to teach us about the children we treat.

I try to invite the teacher's open complaints about the child and maybe the parents. While I don't join the attack, I patiently and nonjudgmentally attend to what she says. I do not have to put the child down in simpatico. I reflect out loud what she says to me. "You've been teaching for 20 years, you say, and you've never seen such a disruptive kid." "You do and do for the family, and all they do is speak badly about you to the principal?" "He seems to want nothing but battle. How frustrating." Or it may simply be my attentive and accepting ear that conveys my sympathy and empathy for her own experience in dealing with the child. Although I probably wouldn't ask it directly, all of my conversation aims to ask the teacher: *What's it like for you* (to teach and be with my patient)? Often the teacher will ask my opinion about something specific. I am wary not to go too fast or offer too much, especially when I am not that sure of what is happening and what is needed.

I'll tell her she's gotten me thinking, which she will have, and I'll thank her for input, making clear my availability (by phone and e-mail) should she wish to talk with me. If, by the call's end, the teacher feels heard, respected, and valued, we have succeeded in getting off to a good beginning.

Readers may be shaking their heads. Who's got time? What psychobabble nonsense? Well, consider what we are attempting to do. Reflect on your own relationships. What makes you feel that your time is valued? What makes you feel that your perceptions and thinking are appreciated? What leads you to want to share your thoughts today and again tomorrow? What makes you care to get more invested? If you answer these candidly, you understand where I'm coming from and why I take such care in my initial interactions with teachers. I further promote our growing connection by encouraging the teacher to contact me with any question, concern, or crisis. Although teachers typically do not use me much in that way and have never abused that open door, they tell me that it is reassuring for them to know that I am there and noticing what they do.

After a couple of weeks, I contact the teacher again, following up on her comments and getting back to her with some reaction to her questions, the seeds of which will evolve into a months-long two-way conversation. I'll refrain from instructing or lecturing, and I'll look for places to intersect what she and I see. "Interesting," I'll say to a teacher who I know dislikes my patient. "He rejects all your help? Boy, that's a real problem 'cause he sure needs a lot of it." Rather than assault her rigidity or ask if she really called him "a moron," I strive to meet her where she

is. "If only we could find a way to get him to want the help he needs."
Most teachers respond to this kind of openness with a blossoming of
empathy and insight. If it seems that I have to be a bit heavier-handed
or direct, I ease down that road. "You know, I'm not sure, but I might
have a hunch as to why he is so allergic to help. Might you want to hear
it?" Now you're asking permission to give an opinion, you say. Yes, I am,
and it works. No one, not me or you, really wants others' advice; it stings
and makes us feel not good enough.

By showing the teacher my empathy, caring, responsiveness, and
respect, she will be more likely to show the child the same in kind. The
more I can listen to her view, the more open she will be to mine. Moreover, teachers are people who care about children. They do not like
feeling disconnected from and unsuccessful with a child. Our buoying
teachers through their difficult and frustrating days with our patients
may enable them to get over the barriers that exist between them and the
child. Over and over I have seen this approach work effectively, helping
to reverse a vicious and downward cycle upward. As the teacher starts to
reach the child, the child will respond, and their constructive relationship
blossoms. Even when the progress is slow and staggering, our confirming and empathic support may be enough to sustain a teacher's optimism
and willingness to keep trying. The modest time we invest in nurturing
that relationship can make us trusting collaborators, giving teachers new
hope and rekindling their greater vision for the child.[1]

The issue of stigma bears mention here. Unlike many, I do not worry
much about the supposed stigma of a child having therapy. In over
25 years of experience, I've never seen one instance where a child was
truly stigmatized by getting help. Such fears, I've found, commonly
belie parents' resistance to the cost, effort, or threat of therapy; parents'
shame or narcissistic injury over having a child who needs treatment;
and, often, greater fears as to whether they or their child is mentally
ill, crazy, beyond help, or dangerous. A sound treatment should never
stigmatize a child. In fact, it should help reduce the child's preexisting
sense of being defective, impaired, or bad, self-perceptions that she has
probably carried alone for some time. I do, however, take the possibility
of stigma seriously when it comes to consulting on the child's behalf.

When talking to schools, I take great care as to the language I use
when referring to the child and her difficulties. I typically steer away from
terms such as "psychotic," "schizophrenic," "borderline," "bipolar," and

"suicidal." These terms tend to evoke stereotypic and simplistic images that take on a life of their own and that can frighten school staff. When teachers use these words, I try to translate them into child's experience. "I'm not sure that she's psychotic. But I know what you mean. When she's stressed, she's prone to take what others say pretty defensively." Teachers will typically respond with concern, making clear that the last thing they ever wish to do is make a child feel bad, no less a child who's susceptible to feeling that way on her own. I occasionally may take a minute or two to discuss the limitations of psychiatric diagnosis. "What I really want to know," I might ask of teachers, "is what you see and think is going on." Being defined as bipolar usually accomplishes little in a school setting. But helping teachers to take a fragile child's perspective can work miracles. We want teachers to know the details of the actual child we treat, not some two-dimensional diagnosis that can short-circuit the more laborious but surer path to getting to know a person.

True enough, there are necessary "moments," meaning deliberative junctures where all the relevant agents, data, and opinions must come together to make a best judgment for the child's educational welfare. Many more times in the course of an academic year, child therapists can proactively help, for instance, preventing small mishaps from turning into major crises or helping a child and a teacher bury a hatchet.[2]

I also am cautious when it comes to communicating with short-term programs, such as summer camps. Parents often don't know whether to "warn" a camp about their child before he gets there. As is true for a majority of clinical decisions, a good rule of thumb is to weigh potential costs against benefits. For example, if a child is doing better in therapy and school, showing increasing signs of self-control and remorse, I will hold back. Why, I figure, should I put a negative idea in someone's head when there's a good chance that the child will do well or, at least, be somewhere in the normal thick of things? Sad to say, self-fulfilling prophecies really do come true. Tell a camp director that Tommy is clinically impulsive or manic, and all of his boyish energy will suddenly loom pathologic and needing intervention.

On the other hand, there are times when programs, like a camp, should know about a child. I've seen many parents who, wanting to not see their child's severe problems, will send him unannounced to a camp, hoping that the lake and sunshine and being around regular kids will undo his troubles. Then, too, there's the issue of false advertising.

I've helped parents to realize that it can be unfair to a camp to "secretly" enroll a child who might be dangerous to himself or other children or whose difficulties will exceed the mission and resources of the camp. But again, as when dealing with schools, I do not sensationalize the child's issues, and I don't rely on psychiatric terms to tell them who the child is. "Tommy can get pretty wild," I might say, adding ways that he has been progressing and approaches that I've found help him to manage himself. And, of course, it's apparent that the child therapist's consulting might include assisting the parent in finding and assessing a camp or activity that suits the child and his developmental needs, especially in the context of his ongoing therapy and advances.

As much as I'd have liked to end the chapter without mentioning legal factors, I can't. It's become an increasingly present and distracting factor for child therapists. What can child therapists do when lawyers, probation officers, or judges come calling? There are cases, we know, when abuse or other horrors demand that therapists be involved legally, filing with social services, for example. Yet I ask *what can clinicians do* purposely, making clear that in a majority of instances child therapists *have a choice*. And choice implies both the privilege and the duty of thinking it through, of making as sound and thorough a clinical judgment as possible.

> Each parent sat in an opposite end of my office, both teary, both enraged. Their two young children wandered the office, anxious and stressed. In spite of an ongoing and angry divorce, we'd tried to do a family meeting, to focus on the issues of the children.
> "She just doesn't get it," the father said, gesturing with disgust.
> "I'm afraid of him," the mother shot back.
> "I know how badly you get along," I reminded them for the ump-teenth time. "But if I distract myself with that, I'll never be able to give the children the help you both want for them."

Both parents felt mistreated, unloved, attacked, and one down. I fully understood their wish for my confirming their perspective. Each wanted me to judge them right and the other wrong. Of course, they would want that.

The case was a tough one just to get going. There was the referral from a psychologist who was trying to negotiate aspects of the extraordinarily messy and traumatic divorce and repeated long calls from the parents, each one telling me why I shouldn't trust the other and wondering how

I thought I could help. It took us over a month of constant e-mails and calls to simply schedule a first meeting.

As we went through this initial phase, each parent had a firm and lengthy list of what they wanted to know from and about me. But I also had my own agenda as to what I wanted them to know about me and how I would proceed with them. I made clear that I was willing to commit to only one thing: doing therapy with the daughter whom they worried about. I also made clear what I would not be doing. I would not, I stated explicitly, be consulting to any aspect of the divorce or custody. I would not write reports or assessments for the court case, and I wouldn't judge or tell a lawyer which one of them was a better parent. I would not question their children about their life at the two parents' homes or which parent they loved better or would rather live with. "All that I can and am willing to do is to do therapy with your child."

As you might guess, the parents begrudgingly agreed. But their behaviors and words pushed me to repeat my vows many times. Whenever either parent contacted me outside of an appointment, their questions about their children always evolved into a scathing attack on the other parent and urged me to take a legal stand on their respective behalf. Time and again, I calmly repeated my original full disclosure that I wouldn't allow my focus on the child to be distracted by the parents' destructive competition. "You need to take your strife to your couples worker and mediator and attorneys," I'd remind them. Gradually, the message sunk in, and the parents' view of me changed. They came to see me as their child's therapist.

Now, I state up front to parents in the midst of a separation or divorce that I will not consult to any legal enterprise. If they seek help for their children, I can offer that. But, I tell them, if they're fishing for evidence, they'd be best off finding themselves a forensic specialist trained and skilled in that area. Most parents hear what I say, confessing that they know their conflicts have harmed and continue to harm their child. Parents occasionally and with embarrassment thank me for my candor and ask if I can refer them to a clinician who can support their legal battle. (A few of these parents have come back to me after the divorce to seek therapy for their child.)

I do not run to talk to judges, lawyers, social services, and the like unless I feel strongly that my doing so will help bring about a beneficial change or prevent one that will be unfavorable to the child's welfare. I've stuck my neck out to advocate for teens and been richly rewarded; I've also been

burned. I have learned to be cautious, not wanting to rescue a delinquent
from consequences that, in the long run, might teach him more and be the
shortest route to the reality testing and growing up he requires. My attitude is fiercely protective of the therapy itself. "Yes, he comes dependably
to his hours" will generally be all that I will share with probation officers
and other agents of the courts and law enforcement.

As we can see, there are varied ways to approach our work as "consul-
tants" to a child's life. Do we proactively intervene, wait and see, or just
plain react? Do we play guru or teammate, director, or adviser? Through
our clinical experience—seeing what works and what doesn't, what brings
benefit and what invokes disaster—child therapists will steadily develop a
firmer sense of and confidence in their preferred style and talents. At the
day's end, however, individual therapists must come to their own judgments
as to what is clinically and ethically called for, ever pursuing what they most
believe will promote the child's best interest at school and elsewhere.

NOTES

1. Who can blame teachers for being wary or reactive to us professionals?
They forever deal with the needs of one or more classrooms of children
while working alongside other teachers, staff, and administrators, under
the not-always-supportive eyes of parents. New regulations and paperwork
never stop coming, and they increasingly are paid less to do more. Imagine
what it must be like for a third-grade teacher to get one of those 27-page
neuropsychology reports that use 45-letter words to describe the child's difficulty adding numbers and that demands eight pages of accommodations,
80 percent of which are impossible at that school. If we really want others,
such as teachers, to understand us and the child, *why do we do things like that?*
And do we really believe that a teacher can do all of that while attending to
24 other children? What are teachers to think?

2. I am not an expert in school consultation. However, here are two
readings that helped me to understand how I might help schools help my
patients. From the vantage point of an educator, Bostic (2001) succinctly
and clearly tells professionals what teachers need from them in order to be
more empowered to work with the child. Sara Lawrence-Lightfoot's *The
Essential Conversation* (2003) lets us into the parent–teacher relationship,
especially as epitomized by the school conference. Her first chapter, "Ghosts
in the Classroom," poignantly reveals how parents' own school experiences
can echo and color their attitude and relationship to their child's education
and teachers.

15

Hard Times: Unwilling Patients and Therapeutic Crises

Few worthwhile enterprises come easy, and child therapy isn't one of them. Pain, doubt, and royal messes tend to accompany almost every substantial course of therapy. That some of our patients find themselves less than enthusiastic about treatment should come as no shock, nor should the fact that many also experience crisis points along the way. This chapter explores both hazards as they apply to child psychotherapy.

UNWILLING PATIENTS

Many onlookers assume that play therapy offers children little more than unbounded play and self-expression under the celebrating eyes of a therapist. Although the kindness, understanding, and tolerance of therapy can be pleasurable—and can themselves be healing and growth advancing—much about child therapy is not at all pleasant for children. Contrary to more naive and devaluing beliefs about our work, child therapists do much more than just play with children. We escort them on their journeys toward self-discovery and self-revision, journeys that often take the child through anguished, humiliating, frightening, uncertain territory. We essentially ask them, no less than our adult patients, to examine themselves—their misbehaviors, their bad attitudes, their greatest anxieties, their deepest and darkest thoughts, their most hidden and precious dreams. Given the awesome nature of what therapy asks of the child, I am struck that more children don't find themselves reluctant to engage in therapy.

"Nice day, isn't it?"
An unusual comment for an 11-year-old boy, it would have been civil enough if it hadn't been the umpteenth time he'd said it this first hour. For that matter, "Nice day, isn't it?" had been the only thing Dana had said for the first 48 or so minutes. Although spoken in a friendly tone with no hint of sarcasm, its being repeated as the answer to questions about himself, his life, and his being here betrayed its resentful purpose: letting me know that Dana did not want to be in therapy.

Wouldn't it have been easier if Dana had just told me that he didn't want to be there? At least we could have talked about that directly. But Dana, understandably, did not feel safe enough with me to share his feeling openly. As it was, and despite himself, he showed some of himself—as we all can't help but do—by expressing his opposition in a passive and seemingly untouchable manner. He had been suspended from school several times and frequently had equivalent difficulties at home, habitually enraging others with superficial gentility that covered much more venomous sentiments. For reasons yet unknown, I knew that Dana did not like doing what others wanted of him.

"Nice day, isn't it?" Dana added one last time in response to my noting that our time was up.
I could have confronted Dana, saying something like, "Don't give me that sweet crap. You don't mean it's a nice day." Or, perhaps, interpreting his behavior à la Hollywood, "You're just a little chicken. You don't have the guts to do therapy. You don't have the balls to talk with me." Who would I have been kidding? Such an outburst would have done nothing therapeutically good, serving mostly to vent my frustration.

"You know, it is a nice day," I replied, meaning it as I opened the door to see the sun shining, reminding myself that Dana's behavior, though aimed at me, was nothing personal about me.

Dana gave me a curious look, my temperance intriguing him. Although he didn't reply, he did come back the next week and the next for many months.

However unique the reasons for Dana's opposition to therapy, he wasn't the only child who sought to avoid therapy with me. I've met exquisitely anxious children for whom the prospect of meeting me, an unknown therapist, to address the very matters that frighten them was itself something very real and big to worry about. More than a few have barricaded themselves in their parents' car in the driveway of my office, refusing to come in. For one of those children, our first four sessions consisted of my standing aside the car, talking through the small crack of the electric window that he controlled while burrowed on the floor under the dashboard. Only after I'd sufficiently demonstrated my patience and respect for his fear and need to control the situation did he dare venture into my office.

Frequently, I find that the children who try to reject therapy from the onset are not anxious enough. These are children, mostly boys, who've been referred because of conflicts with the outside world at home and school. I save my words of how therapy can help them to better understand themselves or live a more fulfilled life. Mistrustful of any authority, they know the score: they've been dragged to me not for self-realization but to fix their badness. Why would any child feel good about seeing a man they assume to be one more arm of the law, a coconspirator who will use his therapeutic disguise to punish and change him?

In some cases my taking an interest in *their* side of the story gets us past their initial guard. Occasionally it does not. In such instances parents often need help and guidance in setting limits on their child's not coming, in finding ways that are firm and effective but do not involve physical aggression or abuse. That some of these homes have been characterized by wrongful uses of force alerts us to be wary, for some parents, if they think we approve, will hog-tie their children to our office. A child who is thrown into our office by the scruff of his neck is unlikely to feel good about us.

Yet occasionally there are children who require behavioral consequences for their lack of cooperation with therapy. These children, from overly lenient homes and headed for delinquency, need discipline and treatment. "Remove the computer from the home until they cooperate with therapy," I've recommended. "Take away their bicycle [or something else that means a lot to them]."

Although children initially detest this idea and its creator (a.k.a. me), they tend to respond well, apparently appreciating at some level that my intervention is in their best interest (because they need discipline and they need treatment) and is a sign of the desperate state their life is in. Once the child is captive in my office, inviting him to openly debate and criticize my opinion helps us to connect and quickly surmount whatever bad feeling was generated by my suggestion. Then and only then can I start to convince children that I am there primarily for them and their needs, however mandated their therapy is. "Any changes you make," I stress, "you'll make because you want to, not because I or anyone else makes you."

Many children balk at or become averse to therapy, as it represents a narcissistic injury. The implication that they may need help offends them, particularly those who most need it. The children who are brought to our door may have been told that they are ill, sick, losers, disturbed, potential serial killers, or have broken brains (which is why we want to know what the child was told about therapy and ourselves and why they are coming). Even in the majority of cases where the words were subtler, gentler, and more tactful, children are apt to read their coming to a mental health professional as announcing their defectiveness or abnormality and signaling their being less than their peers or less than what they or their parents want them to be.

When children tell us, "I don't need your help," they may believe precisely the opposite. But an awareness of their situation or stress may not necessarily translate into a motivation for help. Our telling children that they do need us generally does little more than make them feel yet smaller and more threatened. These children can appreciate our asking them how they figure they've gotten to our doorstep.

> "My asshole father thinks I'm depressed," Geoff said with a disgusted look. "He's the depressed one. He's the one that should be seeing you. I don't need this."
>
> "He really needs to see someone?" I asked back, knowing that Geoff was right, knowing also that his dad actually was in treatment for depression with someone else.

"He does sees someone," Geoff replied, showing me his honesty. "But it doesn't help him."

"No?"

"He walks around like he's going to kill himself any moment."

"You worry about him," I noted, buoyed by Geoff's clear concern for his father, wondering how much his perceptions involved projections of his own suicidal thoughts. The boy's eyes watered.

"I certainly don't know if you're depressed," I said. "You hardly know me, and I hardly know you. But whatever the reasons your parents brought you here, you can make as much or as little of this as you wish."

"Don't think I'm going to talk to you about my feelings and that crap."

"You'll talk about what you want and nothing more."

Geoff proceeded slowly, but gradually he did talk about what he wanted to: what it was like growing up with a father who was so preoccupied with suspicious fears of the world.

I specifically chose to highlight a case in which a boy's reluctance fell by the wayside rather easily and promptly. The majority of children who initially oppose me and the process can be reached with a modest amount of tolerance and the demonstration that I will follow them where they wish to go. I know from experience that a more authoritarian stance, or psychological speculation about the reasons for their fears (even just calling their disinclination toward therapy a fear), can lead them to dig their heels in deeper or flee.

Other children benefit by our demonstrating that we see their wish not to come. We deliberately make statements that include a caboose of a phrase that at least implies that they possibly have an issue that bothers them. "The last thing you want is some therapist poking around your business." "You want to manage your own affairs." "You believe in handling your own troubles." Children who are allergic to help don't want to hear how we will give it to them in some special way. By letting them know that we know they don't want our help, we show them we listen, meet them where they are, confirm and accept their feelings, and testify that our esteem can withstand being unwanted. It also shows children firsthand what therapy is like, how what we offer may be nothing like what they imagine we'll offer and that repels them.

Part of a child's rejection of therapy may reflect mistrust. This suspicion may be well founded following life experiences in which a child had been abused, neglected, or somehow mistreated by a parent or caregiver. As child therapists, we take great care to create an environment and structure that will allay such a child's worries. We willingly keep our doors open (so he can feel in contact with a trusted adult or simply the outside world), conduct therapy with the parent present if the child desires, show him how our doorknobs and locks work (making clear that he can control the comings and goings in the room), and give wide berth to his need for personal space and safety. To children, our proclamations of our trustworthiness mean little and can feel dangerous, whereas our announcement of our understanding for their caution ("After all, you know nothing about me except that I'm a therapist") and support for their getting to know us slowly does much to allay their protective reservations concerning therapy and us.

Children who have grown up in more sociopathic homes may distrust our motives. They may think that therapists are self-serving. They assume we do our work solely for love of money and have no true caring for them or their families. Our statements that we do care about them and their welfare fall on deaf ears, for they have learned that such claims are the manipulating tongue of con men. They may ask questions that test us severely but that we can't afford to duck. "If you care so much about me, why don't you see me for free?" Although to answer, "Of course I would," may feel good to us, it's probably not true and risks confirming the hunch that we are liars. Our being straight with them and exhibiting our caring over time is the only antidote to their cynicism.

The dependency of therapy can make children uncomfortable and lead them to withhold their attachment and investment in treatment and the therapist. Essentially dreading saying good-bye, they can never bring themselves to say hello. An unfair irony tends to rule in this matter. Those whose dependency needs are strongest commonly push others away the hardest, including the child therapist. These children, self-declared islands, find the nurturing shelters we create seductive but perilous. They know, even in their short lives, that others can't be counted on to be there, not to die, not to neglect, not to abuse, not to abandon. Only fools, they are sure, grow reliant on others. Such children may be hardened and cold-shouldered to humanity or may have turned wholly to peers for the support and affiliation they crave. We make contact with these children slowly.

Passed among a chaotic and dysfunctional extended family because no one, including his parents, had the resources to care for him adequately and consistently, nine-year-old Vincent had come to depend on his own wits to get by. The social agency that managed his case had referred him to me for escalating aggression at school.

Vincent needed nobody. He told me so often in our beginning work. "No thanks," he said, politely declining my offer for a snack. He readily deflected my questions concerning his comfort (e.g., wanting more heat or fresh air). "Whatever you want," he'd reply. He was perfectly polite and willing to discuss whatever I brought up, but I felt as though I was an annoying fly that Vincent calmly brushed off again and again. (In fact, I'd seen Vincent deal with a bee in the office exactly that way, showing that he could care less about the insect, even as he chased it away.) "I have no needs," every word and gesture seemed to protest. "I'm okay with what I've got."

Several weeks into our meetings, Vincent arrived with a bad cold. The dryness of the office caused him to cough. "Can I get you some water?" I asked, watching his clear discomfort. He held up his hand to signal no while struggling with a coughing jag that wouldn't end. Putting his physical need above the psychological one not to need, I brought him out a tall glass of water with a handful of hard candies. Still gagging, he took the water while holding up his hand to ward off the candy. A couple of sips did the trick, and, the water barely touched, Vincent promptly put the glass on the table alongside the candy and thanked me. "It's awfully dry in here," I said, wanting to put the responsibility of his need on the environment (as if to say, "It's not your fault you needed water in here" and, going one step further, "it's not your fault you have needs"). Trivial as this act of giving and taking may seem, Vincent reacted severely. He grew more defiant at school—he'd settled down a bit since treatment—and withdrew even more in therapy, discussing neither his rejuvenated problems nor anything else.

The therapy barely thumped along until one day Vincent came to a session soaked from a thunderstorm. (Dressing for the weather would be admitting his needs to himself.) I offered to get him a towel.

"Fuck you!" he responded, cursing at me for the first time. Vincent looked away. I tried inquiring what might be bothering him: school, home, friends. But my words didn't touch him. I was stymied. Watching him dry his drenched head with a small piece of tissue he had, however, brought the light to me.

"You never asked for that water, did you?" I asked.

"What!" Vincent snapped, though I was certain he'd heard me.

"You never asked that for that water, did you?"

"I didn't ask for it and I didn't need it."

"I just brought it, didn't I?"

"I don't need any fucking thing from you. Or anybody else." Vincent's eyes reddened. We spent the remainder of the hour in silence.

Although he had a much better week at school following that hour and soon after spontaneously asked me where those hard candies had gone, Vincent's fear of depending on me and people, while shrinking considerably, dogged every last inch of his therapy.

Needing not to need me, Vincent kept me at bay. A child's begrudging attitude, expressed notably in terms of criticism of the therapist, however, can carry meaning beyond that of fearing dependency.

Karin couldn't get along with anyone. She alienated her family, teachers, and peers. "He doesn't help me," she declared loudly, even in the initial hour, lobbying her parents to be excused from treatment. "I'm never going to talk with him," she promised them, though her wish to put me down moved her to speak continually. "You're stupid," she told me minutes later. She also informed me that I was ugly, boring, pathetic, queer, dishonest, and a complete waste of space.

Karin's name-calling didn't bother me, for it was easy to feel her presence and caring. But the tirades gradually faded, and Karin spent more of each hour in quietude, with eyes closed and arms crossed, determined not to share any work with me. "He does me no good," she'd announce at the hour's end. "I don't even talk in there." Fortunately, her parents, feeling so at their rope's end, had no intention of stopping therapy however much she complained.

"It's perplexing," I said, during Karin's silence. "Your life's in a shambles. You're here anyway. And yet you stubbornly refuse to give it a try."

"For what?" Karin angrily came back. "I've been coming for two months, and you haven't helped me yet."

"You haven't tried."

"I've come for weeks, and my life's as screwed up as it ever was. You can't help me. No one can."

Karin's need to devalue me and therapy came, I soon learned, from her sense of utter hopelessness that no one could ever help her and make her life any different, any better. Establishing this despair together allowed the therapy to begin in earnest.

In most cases our child patients' reluctances in treatment reflect resistances that involve the therapeutic work itself rather than the therapist's failure to engage them. Their misgivings are not aimed at us personally; that is, they are not resisting us as individuals. They resist looking at themselves honestly out of fear of what they might see. For example, one boy preferred blaming his not skiing on his mother's overprotectiveness rather than acknowledging his own fear of injury and loss of control. None of us, including our child patients, wish to see parts of ourselves that tarnish our ideal images of who we are and who we want to become.

The benefit of clear self-vision, stressed throughout this book and continually demonstrated in our clinical work, is easier to grasp for some children. Consider a child whose bad-boy cruelty hides a strong underlying wish to be a good and caring child. Who would argue that his coming to see, accept, and take pride in that part of himself is anything but wonderful? What other children see in the mirror, however, may be less appreciated by families or society.

Mae was the sweetest of daughters. This 10-year-old was generous, nurturing, and considerate to a fault. An honors student and always the first to help out, she was every teacher's favorite. When others fought, she made peace. If it were not for the severe headaches and stomach pains for which she was referred, her life, her parents reported, would be perfect.

For many hours in therapy, Mae showed herself to be the model citizen I'd been told about, concerned only for others' welfare, taking care of my office and me as much as she could. During one migraine attack, however, she expressed a smidgen of frustration over the noise of children in the waiting room. I was watching to see if that small venting of hostility might alleviate her headache, but it only worsened it. "I'm sorry," she said, near tears. "I'm just not feeling well."

"They are noisy, aren't they?" I concurred. "It could give anyone a headache, don't you think?" Now her face relaxed, and a smile broke out. My tolerance and the sharing of her plaint comforted her and eased her pain.

Over her course of treatment, Mae grew much more able to disagree and protest. As she became more open to making claims for her own needs, she was no longer the perfect little lady. While pleased that her bodily pains subsided, her parents were more ambivalent about the daughter she was becoming. She now fought with her family, occasionally had tensions with her teachers, and was not nearly as selfless as she once was. They appreciated Mae's becoming a more confident person who could assert her ideas, and they highly valued her becoming more able to protect herself even if it meant hurting another's feelings. Her fortified independence toward them, however, was much harder for them to adapt to and occupied much of Mae's worry and work on her way to growing up.

Looking at oneself honestly can be starkly lonely and pained. One boy may not like admitting that he wants to be an only child, for that, in his good-boy's mind, would make him his little sister's murderer. One girl may not want to know how badly she wishes she was a boy, fearing its homosexual meanings and, even more, not wanting to feel the sad hopelessness of that never-to-come-true fantasy. Another child may not like discovering just how devoted he is to being angry with his mother, believing that to let it go would be to wholly pardon her. For many adolescent boys, their wish to be taken care of in therapy evokes terrifying homophobia. The reasons none of us want to look ourselves in the eye are complex, deep, and substantial.

While a child's resistance can manifest itself suddenly or in highly discrete moments, it much more often permeates the entire fabric of a therapy, rising and falling in different contexts and under varying stresses. This resistance does not avert unwanted insights per se as much as it wards off the demand for change that awareness brings. If a boy admits that he is selfish, he then bears the responsibility of staying selfish or becoming more generous.

If I'm hostile, do I want to stop fighting and hurting people? If my insecurity leads me to put down other children, am I willing to treat them better? If I am afraid of everything, am I willing to take risks to conquer my worry? Whatever the precise form of a child's resistance, it may involve some variation on the wish to never grow up. That is why the lag between significant insights and behavioral changes can be great and discouraging—to the child, his parents, and the therapist. General resistance to the losses and responsibilities of growing up is at the core, I have found, of almost every treatment.

As we know too well, parents' resistance is an equally likely obstacle to our work with their child.

Mrs. Newman loved her son dearly. She was a single mother and he an only child. For better and worse, they enjoyed an embattled, enmeshed, and overly intimate relationship. Having brought Harry in with a growing depression, she felt much genuine appreciation that therapy was working, which is why I was caught off guard by her last-minute canceling of three sessions in a month's period. "He's sick," "I'm sick," and "He has too much schoolwork to get done for tomorrow" were the messages she left (contrasting with her typically friendly tone).

"Sick?" Harry asked, when I asked about his health on his return. Harry explained that he'd missed sessions because his mother took him to buy a bicycle in lieu of the first missed session, took him to a movie instead of his second, and invited him to skip school the morning of the third with the provision that he not leave the house all day.

I didn't have to hit Mrs. Newman on the head with my finding that she'd lied. To do so would have humiliated her, put Harry in an impossible place, and thrown the therapy off track. Instead, I shared with Mrs. Newman my realization of how hard it can be to bring a child to a therapist.

This simple statement of empathy tapped a torrent of emotions: fear that I would steal her son away, dread that I was the parent she wished she could have been, jealousy that her son's treatment was working better than her own, and a pained conviction that she caused him hurt (i.e., depression) but that I healed him. "Do you know what it's like to feel like you have to bribe your own child to make him like you more?" she asked, in all of the anguish a parent can feel, confessing and interpreting in that awful question all that she'd done the past month. Mrs. Newman and I made a deal that day, one that she kept, that should she feel that I was growing too close to her son, she would take me to task (with words).

Most parents feel bad when their child suffers or has sufficient troubles to need a therapist. Few parents celebrate their child's coming for treatment. The changes that the child undergoes may force changes at home; such disequilibriums in the family as a whole are at the heart of family systems treatments. The child's being in therapy and the matters that inevitably arise confront parents. Hard reality may clash with their ideals of the parents they wanted to be and the dreams they held for their children. Beyond the obvious narcissistic injury, these realizations can cause profound heartache and despair.

As underlined in the previous chapter on parent work, we must always keep watch for signs of such resistance. We try to prevent these doubts from growing too large lest parents end treatment. We encourage them, making clear their obligation, to share their frustrations with us. We don't let too many no-shows or last-minute cancellations pass before trying to understand them and do something constructive. Rather than defensively justify the costs and effort of therapy, we try to understand the sacrifice parents are making as well as their resentment. We also consider the possible red herrings their protests may pose as we listen for the basic ambivalence toward their child that may underlie them.[1]

THERAPEUTIC CRISES

We all know a crisis when we see one: a person stands on the edge of a bridge, or threatens someone with a steak knife, or violently assaults another, or swallows a bottle of medication. I leave the discussion of those horrors to another book, another author. In this section I discuss what I call *therapeutic crises*, meaning junctures or phases in a sound and ongoing therapy where there is: deterioration of symptoms, behaviors, or functioning; a disturbing lack of progress; heightened (or newly surfaced) self-destructive impulses; or a serious narcissistic blow to our child patients or their parents.

> I looked at the family before me. Mr. and Mrs. Isley appeared as deeply stressed as their son, Leo, who'd been in treatment with me for the past year and a half. Although Leo's anxiety and timidity had diminished dramatically during the first 11 months, he'd gone downhill since. His school, which had cheered his blossoming, was calling again with concerns over just how tense and unable to function this fifth grader was. "What can we do?" the parents asked, just as they'd asked so many times before.
>
> Following a sudden profit in the stock market a couple of years earlier, the Isleys had bought a massive estate along the riverfront. Although Mr. Isley had no regular job or income, that windfall had convinced him of future good fortune and attested to his giftedness as an investor. But the times had turned down fast. Greed and impulsivity had led Mr. Isley to make several bad decisions that cost them most of their savings. Facing the possibility of bankruptcy, Mr. Isley had begun drinking (an old problem for him), as had Mrs. Isley.
>
> When we met, they discussed the overwhelming stress that their mortgage payment was having on them. "If we just sold the estate," they explained repeatedly, "we could buy an extremely nice home and have a good deal of savings. Less stressed, we could function better,

find ourselves jobs." They looked at Leo. "And we know this is killing the kids."

I nodded my head in agreement.

Although I proceeded to make clear my agreement that the stress was killing all of them and that the resurgence of alcoholism would only complicate matters, I was handcuffed. They understood the impact their financial situation was having on themselves and their family, yet losing that property and all that it meant was almost impossible for them.

Tempted to give up, I continued. The fact that the Isleys continued to come signaled at least some ambivalence, and I stayed true to my child patient. Leo still needed my help to stay afloat in this overwrought family but eventually found himself able to confront his parents on their selfishness and how it was destroying him. It was his doing so that moved them to take the action that was long overdue, that did bring them much of the relief and hope they'd imagined.

There have been other families, however, whom I have been unable to reach in this way and from whom I actually resigned.

"I know it's the weekend, but I'm really afraid for Kent."

Hearing this message, I called Mrs. Thiessen. She described how eight-year-old Kent had stolen again. We scheduled an appointment for Sunday morning.

Mrs. Thiessen told me how Kent had stolen a pocketbook from their neighbor. I was bothered by the fact that he'd deliberately planned the crime on the day this kindly widow, a woman who was good to him, cashed her Social Security check. But I wasn't shocked: this young child from an affluent home had stolen many times before. He lied habitually and blamed others. His character, sad to say, was quite flawed.

For at least the third time, we discussed a fitting punishment. Mr. and Mrs. Thiessen thought their disapproval should be sufficient even though this was becoming a repetitive problem. I suggested that Kent be made to work for two hours each afternoon for 50 cents an hour until he'd earned back all of the money plus interest. The parents, worried about his becoming a sociopath, agreed enthusiastically.

Several weeks later, however, I received another frantic call: Kent had stolen again. While sharing their upset about this new incident, the parents made clear their displeasure with my inquiring about the previous one. "How was that discipline going?" I asked, having received a note from them that "it seemed to be having an effect" on Kent. With some prodding I learned that Kent had done no work. "We just don't have any work that a child can do at our house," Mr. Thiessen declared. "And besides, what do you expect me to do? Stand there for an hour a day watching to make sure he works?"

To make a long story short, I eventually resigned from the case, making it clear that I could not help Kent, that talking with me would bring him no benefit as long as his dishonest and scheming behavior was minimized and tolerated. With his parents neither willing to do what was needed nor willing to examine their reasons for that apathy, my play and talking cure was useless.

One of the commonest therapeutic crises is when old symptoms recirculate and return with a vengeance.

Andy's parents had brought her to therapy because of her uncontrollable tantrums. But over the past year she'd grown much in her capacity to tolerate frustration and to accept limitations. The birth of a new sister, however, brought her tantrums back with explosive force. "We can't take her anymore," her mother tearfully confessed.

My helping Andy's mother remember the gains her daughter had made, while confirming her frustration (particularly her being overwhelmed by new motherhood), steadied the home front a bit. My putting Andy's regression into a developmental context and predicting its passage was enough to settle Andy's mother, who feared not so much today's or tomorrow's tantrum but that those difficulties would go on forever.

Parents' impulsive decisions to stop therapy can often indicate a crisis, as it did with Austin.

"This is Mrs. Bates. Austin won't be coming for therapy anymore. Thanks for all your help. Just send us the last bill, and we'll pay you immediately."

Mrs. Bates had never felt close to me, but her unexpected message was even colder than I'd considered her to be. Given how beautifully her 12-year-old son, Austin, had done in therapy—brought because of pervasive inhibition due to a dog phobia that followed his having been bitten—her bulletin frankly shocked me. I wondered what I might have said or done to offend her but couldn't come up with anything.

I waited a few days, hoping that whatever was burning might have cooled, and called her. She didn't want to talk, but when I expressed fear that I'd somehow let *her* down, she opened up. Mrs. Bates told me with fury how, when she entered the bathroom during her son's bath, Austin had pushed her out, telling her he wanted privacy. The kicker was when he told her that he hated her.

"But he's doing much better now, isn't he?" I said naively.

"I don't care how he's doing. I'd rather have him depressed. I'm not going to tolerate any son of mine saying that he hates me."

I was horrified that a mother could say that about her own child. But I reminded myself, "Wasn't it she who brought him to therapy?" Besides, it hit me, hadn't therapy taken off, not when he played out dog attacks but when he connected his fear of dogs and his fear of his mother, a woman who could be cruelly intimidating? Supervising myself, I responded more suitably. "You bring your son for therapy, and what do you get for it?" I asked Mrs. Bates, hoping she'd let me back in.

And she did. For Mrs. Bates, like any mother who loves her son, didn't want to be hated by him. While I saw Austin's hatred as expressing the other side of his deep love, an expression that would make room for them to grow even closer, she heard only hatred that in her worst nightmares would grow and grow until he'd want nothing to do with her ever. Yet more than many mothers, Mrs. Bates had some sense that how she'd treated her son had given him good reason to hate her.

When parents threaten the end of therapy, we must take their thinking seriously. What might be triggering their upset, we ask ourselves? Our own retaliative and impulsive urge to find out fast, to alleviate our own worries (that it isn't something we'd done), or to convince them otherwise is paradoxically the longest way around. Slow and steady is the course, leaving ample room for parents and ourselves to wallow in and come to better know what good reasons are making them doubt whether therapy is in their child's best interest. Almost without exception, parents' abrupt decisions to terminate therapy signal that something important is afoot, something that must be tracked down and reckoned with, not just to renew the therapy but to resolve a matter that likely holds significance for the child and parent as well as the treatment.

Perhaps the most difficult of therapeutic crises is when a child expresses a wish to die. This wish may make itself known in a passing bedtime utterance: "I wonder what the point of living is?" It can come more dramatically, during a frustrated homework moment: "I hate myself. I'm so stupid. I wish I'd just die." Or it can be observed in endless sobbing, accompanied by hopelessness, helplessness, and sometimes cruel self-deprecating. Such distress is never easy to see or hear. For a loving parent to hear a child wish himself dead is beyond painful.

"Rick can't stop crying," his mother, who'd asked for this hour, told me with her own wet eyes. She held her head in her hands.

"What is it?" I asked

"What did I do," she asked herself in my presence, barely able to get the words out, "to make my baby hate himself?"

I sat and said nothing, allowing Rick's mother to cry all she needed. She didn't need me to answer this question, to give her a laundry list of parenting faults and missteps. Nor did I rush to undo the guilt she felt. My job was to stay with her in the awful place she found herself.

At the hour's end I explained what I knew for sure. Rick had been doing better than ever. Once thoroughly depressed and dysfunctional, he was living life. He had become an active and successful member of his classroom. He'd made a couple of friends even if he still hung back socially. Depressive bodily symptoms had improved: eating again, he'd gained 12 pounds; he could fall asleep in less than an hour versus the several he used to require; and he had become a somewhat avid bike rider.

Once much too depressed and forlorn to discuss his obvious suffering—including the traumatic loss of a father who, when Rick was four, had left town and his son for good—Rick had grown strong enough to feel his hurt and to share it. "Rick," I explained, "is feeling good enough to finally withstand that sadness."

"You mean his crying is a good thing?" his mother asked with hope in her eyes.

I readily nodded my affirmation, knowing that what she'd said was exactly the way it was.

In a majority of cases, when child patients who are firmly ensconced in therapy with me talk of death and hating themselves, I find myself encouraged, sometimes elated. For months, usually years, these children have, all alone, carried their horrid sense that they are bad, sick, evil, crazy, or worse. The boy who can finally tell his parents and his therapist of these sentiments has come a long way in trust, resiliency, and hope. He feels good enough about himself to think that another person will care about his hurt. He feels optimistic enough to believe that sharing his hurt will bring some relief or consolation. He's come to recognize that shedding these weighty thoughts can bring a lightness not known before. Ironically, his sharing these thoughts generally means that he is not so persuaded that he is in fact as disturbed, insane, or worthless as he once judged himself to be.

While scary thoughts can lead us to fear for the child's welfare, we may also worry about legal matters and our liability. It is imperative that we try to keep those needs distinct from what transpires and is warranted clinically. Hospitals occasionally can keep children safe, but in general not much happens therapeutically. Children are typically released in much the same state as they were admitted, ready now to begin the outpatient therapy that has been unnecessarily delayed.

Of course, children who are in danger, who are trying to kill themselves or hurt others, need to be protected. However, when a child is working steadily in a productive therapeutic relationship, verbal expressions of self-hatred and suicide and even milder acts of self-destruction can often be best left in the trusting, hopeful, and holding hands we offer them.

We, as therapists, firmly hold our child patients and their parents through this necessary misery on the road to recovery and healing. But we can only do so when we truly believe that what we are seeing is a good sign. We strive at these trying times to see clearly the context of the child's life and therapy. Fitful crying jags or suicidal ideation in themselves say little about the prognosis or how serious things are. I have yet to see any serious therapy, with child or adult, not come to moments of existential doubt. To live a thinking life is, I believe, to have times of utter despair and questions as to the purpose and value of life. The more closely and carefully we follow children and their therapy from the initial steps across our threshold, the more likely we are to understand and know how to handle the inevitable crises that evolve in the course of this tumultuous work.[2]

Even the most skilled and successful of therapies is prone to obstacles, detours, and crises. These seeming impasses need not be signs of the patient's deterioration or the therapist's negligence (though they can be, of course). To the contrary, in a well-founded treatment relationship they often speak to points of opportunity that, if appreciated in their unique context, can richly facilitate a therapy and bring greater understanding not just to those patients but to all of our clinical work.

NOTES

1. Books dedicated to engaging difficult children: Richard Gardner (1990) proposes various interventions to work with the resistant child. Meeks and Bernet (2001) spotlight the fragile alliance that can exist between

adolescents and their therapists. Finally, my own and recent book (Bromfield, 2005) explores ways that therapists can help their teen patients take ownership of and responsibility for their therapies and, more so, their lives.

2. Consider Hoffman and Remmel's (1975) paper on crisis intervention. They break a crisis into initial, middle, and termination phases and see the creation of an empathic milieu as key to enabling the child to express himself and his crisis (uncovering the *why now?*). Terr et al.'s (2005) paper on "moments" in therapy is also revealing, as she and colleagues see each therapy as having a story of its own and a plot that includes critical turning points or moments of truth.

16

Getting to Know You, Getting to Know Me: Race, Religion, and Culture

C hild therapy is about forming relationships with other people and intimately understanding their experiences and perspectives. How can the child's and therapist's race, religion, and culture not be relevant? Of course, this chapter cannot substitute for in-depth study of these issues. Nor will it focus on any one people. It will, I hope, provoke clinicians to revisit big ideas that may seem too obvious to write about and to consider some new and counterintuitive possibilities for their work with children and families.

Cultural difference can make an impact very early in our work with a child and a family. One family taught me this early in my private practice. When the referring agency hadn't been able to find a Khmer-speaking clinician, I'd agreed to test a young Cambodian boy who lived in the poorest neighborhood of a poor city. I anticipated the meeting with worry. How, with our language differences, would I ever conduct a decent testing? My telephone call with the father quelled my fear.

Despite some mutual confusion, he seemed to get the directions to my home and office.

Not knowing how long the testing might take, I'd set aside an entire Saturday afternoon. But dinner and darkness came, and they hadn't shown. I closed my office and put away the testing materials, frustrated at having lost a gorgeous fall day and knowing I'd have to reschedule. As my family set down for dinner, at least six hours past the scheduled appointment, we heard a noisy vehicle pull into the driveway. I ran outside to see a kindly and tired man, the boy's father, who apologized profusely for having gotten so lost, more than a 100 miles into the neighboring state. I met the boy only after his mother, both sets of grandparents, an elderly great-grandparent, an aunt and uncle, and several siblings climbed out of the van. I offered them something to eat, but they politely deferred, showing me that they'd brought along bags and a cooler of food they'd made for the day. As I watched the caravan of family move into my office, I looked at my clock. It was almost 7:00. How would this clinical misadventure ever come to a good end?

But it did. With my insistence over their polite objections, we reorganized the furniture in my waiting room to create a comfortable space for them to eat and relax. Several of the adults asked to come in the office to watch the testing, something I'd never done before. But the boy wanted that, too. With a small audience behind me, we began the testing. It quickly became clear to me that our inability to speak each other's language would severely limit the assessment. However, I again was proven wrong. The uncle deftly served as translator, knowing when to say just enough to make my directions understood. Quietly and without intrusion, the family watched, not to scrutinize me but to support the boy they adored and wanted only the best for. Having spent their day in a van, stressed over being lost and missing their appointment, this family was nothing but smiles and appreciation.

Yes, it turned out to be a happy ending. The boy was very bright and scored high, his superior abilities to think and problem solve pronouncing themselves loudly. When they left, near midnight and some 14 hours after they'd left their home, my office smelling deliciously of curry and coconut, the boy and his family, each and everyone of them, thanked me, a gratitude they showed me again by mailing me a copy of his acceptance letter to a school for gifted children. And yet the pleasure and the thanks was more my own. This family had given me a profound lesson in humility, patience, respect, and love of family. Their wondrous presence in my tiny waiting room had forced me to rethink every preconception I held about clinical work. It reminded me of what my services can mean to a child and family and to never take that responsibility lightly or glibly.

In order for us to continue this chapter together, it is only fair and necessary that I now disclose who I am. It probably won't surprise any reader to hear that I am a white, relatively nonreligious Jewish man of Russian descent who grew up in a working-class city of Massachusetts where I was educated in public schools, a private college, and a state university. How much does this matter? Well, as you will see, enough to make me need to think and learn plenty. Your knowing, I suspect, might also help you to understand blind spots or biases of mine that jump out at you as you read this chapter or maybe that you've already observed in earlier chapters. Does my heritage, race, and background impair my work? Probably no more or less than yours or any other therapist's does. And, as we'll soon discover together, when it comes to understanding and connecting with our patients, who we are can be as much a blessing as a curse.

As a graduate student at the University of North Carolina, I worked with African American children from the inner city and from poor, rural areas. I thought I was rather prejudice free, and to some degree I was. But these children and families, again, showed me much to the contrary, children like Russell, a six-year-old boy who was as learning disabled as he was handsome and athletic. Russell and I connected quickly. He loved sports, and so did I. He loved to play, and so did I. He wanted help, and I wanted to give it. We both ran to our meetings, and we both hated when the time was up. So what was the problem?

Russell's mother seemed not to share any of her son's good feeling for me and the treatment. She shunned my overtures and declined my invitations to meet. She avoided me at all costs, dropping off and picking up Russell at the curb front of the community clinic where we met. I naively made the worst of it, misreading all of its meaning, believing that Russell's mother didn't support his therapy and that she wasn't doing all she could to help. It wasn't until the final hour of our year together that, as we say in New England, dawn broke over Marblehead.

Russell and I had said our sad good-byes, and we headed toward the clinic door. His mother stood outside her car. She held a bouquet of flowers. With tears in her eyes and welcoming her son to her side with the biggest hug I'd ever seen, she handed the flowers to me. My sight renewed, I wanted to say it all—how sorry I was for giving her an occasional hard time, for thinking anything but the best of her, and for missing the most obvious truth of all: that she'd brought Russell to see me week after week, rain or shine, and even the week of a once-in-a-century snowstorm that hit Chapel Hill that year. That, more than anything she could have said, was the proof positive of her love and caring for her son. But it was way too late for all that. We just said good-bye.

What have I done differently with parents since? I never forget that bringing one's child for help is almost always a loving and caring act. When a parent, particularly one of color, avoids me, I don't get sidetracked by taking it personally. Instead, I presume they have good reason for not wanting to meet or work with me. Rather than punish or hammer them, I respect that need or decision. More often than not, that acceptance leads to eventual closeness and my learning what that reservation or mistrust is about. Why would a mother whose been mistreated by outside agencies trust me? She'd be a fool to. Why would an African American man whose grown-up enduring racism toward his parents, himself, and maybe his children feel good about me, a white stranger? No good reason I've yet to think of. I now acknowledge it directly. "Given what you've been through, it must be so hard to bring your daughter to me and this place." "You have no obligation to like or trust me. Only my behavior as we get to know one another will show you who I really am." I have yet to meet any person of any color who doesn't respond to this candid reality. And, I agree, in retrospect I would not think it too late to have told Russell's mother about my missteps and to express my regret that I'd misunderstood her and missed out being able to help her more. She deserved as much.

The concept of therapy itself, we must keep in mind, is not a universal that's shared by all people. Where I grew up in Revere, a working-class city north of Boston, no one I knew saw a therapist. On Long Island, where my wife grew up, a lot of people did. Are people in New York crazier? Probably not. Their idea of going to talk with another person, maybe even doing it while lying on a couch, is much less foreign, more familiar, and likely more acceptable than it is in many other parts of the country. So, even when we know we can help another person, it doesn't necessarily mean that they will embrace us and that possibility. Taking help from professionals is not second nature to some groups. There are cultures in which seeing a medicinal herbalist or religious shaman would be considered more conventional and reasonable than going to a psychotherapist. Some Eastern cultures find American psychology to be a limited and selfish perspective, reflecting what they view as our society's unhealthy preoccupation with the individual, her feelings, achievements, and satisfaction. In fact, they might describe our psychotherapy as not a remedy but an essential symptom of what is wrong with our way of life. And lots of immigrant groups, new and old, not to mention many descendants of the Pilgrims and Puritans, see personal feelings and family life as private and not to be aired in either the laundry or the therapy room.

Rather than reflect simple resistance, the reasons that parents are against their child's therapy can be large and reveal significant aspects of their culture and way of viewing the world, as it was for Gani, an 11-year-old boy from Turkey and the son of two scientists. Although Gani was very anxious and had experienced a major trauma, his parents brought him to me only because they felt pressured to by a schoolteacher whom they thought highly of. Our first few meetings were wholly occupied with Gani's parents asking me many questions about therapy and how it worked, each of which they debated in the negative. Their fears were substantial and steeped in their upbringing. While they didn't like seeing the distress that their son's perfectionism caused him, they worried that therapy might weaken his unrelenting ambition and make him too comfortable with himself, make him "American lazy." They also wanted him to learn to handle life, a skill that they believed therapy and its dependency could undermine. Their own tough lives had taught them the value of resiliency, and they were determined not to cheat Gani out of his. After several meetings, we agreed that they would be most comfortable using me then not as a therapist but as a parenting consultant, integrating my insights into their home in ways that made sense to them. My respecting their perspective made for a good experience that, as I've often found happens, keeps the door open should they someday want or need more help.

Sometimes as child therapists, we meet people whose religious views are set firmly against what we do. I've worked with several fundamentalist families, Christian and Jewish, who come to me only because they feel they have no other choice.

"He just needs his faith renewed." That's what Michael's father told me in our first meeting. "He really doesn't need this psychology stuff."

I didn't contest what Michael's father had said. Michael's parents, I knew, had tried several Christian counselors who'd given up, who'd told them that their only son was mentally ill, maybe schizophrenic, and who'd referred them elsewhere. Michael's parents had come to me as a last resort, in the same way that they'd enrolled him in a public school after his religious school said they could no longer handle him. Their reluctance, I had then thought, went beyond their faith to their wish that the son they loved was just lost and not seriously ill. I didn't challenge their faith; I rarely do. Their faith, moreover, was about the only certainty in a family of alcoholism, verbal abuse, unreliability, great marital conflict, and parents who were themselves deeply unhappy.

"My parents think what you do is crazy. They pray for you," Michael told me.
"They do?" I asked.
"All the time," Michael replied.

By that time, I knew Michael well enough to know that he wasn't trying to provoke me. He was confused by his parents' belief that I needed their praying. Talk about a bind! Three previous therapists had judged Michael to be too ill for them to help. Those who knew best were telling him something worrisome about the therapist, so he thought, who was actually helping him. As readers might imagine, questioning authority, especially his parents, was dangerous. Michael's therapy was headed toward helping him to recognize his lack of faith, not in God but in his own perceptions.

"My head's going to explode." Michael pulled his hair. "I don't know what to believe," he said. "It's tearing me apart."

Michael was better. His tyrannical self-hatred had diminished as had his persecutory hallucinations and his once diagnosed Tourette's. His suicidal impulses had ceased, and he had begun to make friends at school. So why was Michael torn? As he'd improved, he'd gained confidence in his own thoughts and feelings. His parents weren't pleased. They transferred Michael from his public school to a Christian academy where they told him to beware of Jews who, like wolves in sheep's clothing, disguise their evil behind kind and helpful pretenses. The message was too much for Michael. His experience told him that I hadn't been doing the devil's work, and yet he wondered and worried whether I was. Michael's parents took his growing conflict and doubts about me as a sign to pull him out of treatment with me and to give Christian therapy another try. I had no option but to abide by their decision and made clear my availability should they ever change their minds.

When very religious parents ask me whether I'll accept their or their child's faith, I answer forthrightly that I look at faith in much the same way I look at other aspects of a child's or family's life. I respect it as a choice. If the child, however, wants to question that faith, I wholly support that work. If a parent's religious practices or intolerance are burdening their child, I have to say so. Unlike Christian counselors, I do not see lack of faith as a cause of mental illness. Nor do I see renewing their faith as the road to better health and adjustment.

In working with Orthodox Jews, I often have found myself walking the same tightrope, wanting to do my best to help a child who hurts but needing to offer that help within the context of the family's strong and long-standing faith and tradition. As clinicians, we strive to help the child live and thrive within the home and culture that is their own. I do not, for example, advise Orthodox parents to loosen up and let their child trick-or-treat on Halloween. I do, however, work hard to create an open space in which children of Orthodox homes (or any other) can themselves wonder, explore, and complain about the demands and restrictions of their religion. Should a child want to lobby their parent for a cheeseburger or some other forbidden taste, I try to help them understand their frustration and wishes in the larger context. Should they, the children, want to question their beliefs with their parents and should they want my support for that, I give it, making clear to parents that the thinking came from the child. I further spotlight the importance of valuing that self-reflection, whatever its effect on the child's spiritual commitment. And, just as I'd welcome any gift a child brings, I celebrate and confirm the aspects of their religious faith that brings them comfort and joy, for how can such things ever be bad?

Perhaps curious to some, these questions of faith in therapy apply not only to formal religions but to other forms of spirituality. We try to honor families' beliefs even as we allow ourselves to wonder about them and sometimes even to query. I don't believe we can talk to the dead, but several of my patients' parents do. I suspect that, if we are willing to hear it, many more people than we realize believe it also. I try to understand their sentiments, wanting more so to learn how these beliefs affect the home and the child who may or may not share them. I do not laugh or roll my eyes at their interest in the paranormal. If I do so, that will be the last time they share anything precious with me. If there's anything I know, it's that these children and parents are trying their best to understand and cope with a life that, if anything, is hard, uncertain, and full of hurt and disappointment. I likewise treat atheism as a belief to be heeded and pondered. What, I listen for, are the antecedents to their lack of faith. Does their atheism soothe them, trouble them, or neither? Is their atheism well founded, or does it reflect an inability to commit, surrender, love, or need others? Deep devotion or utter existentialism, Muslim or Buddhist, they are all the same to me as a clinician—to be heeded, understood, and sometimes probed.

Increasingly we meet children whose parents are of different races or religions. Is this cause for a different kind of concern or intervention? The answer is mostly no, of course, with a proviso. What, we have to ask ourselves as clinicians, are the implications, if any, for the child? When a child is torn between fighting parents, it is always a bad thing. It can be yet more confusing when a child's beliefs are torn between warring parents who want the child to believe what they believe and reject what the other parent believes. In my experience, children can grow up to love who they are when their parents can do the same and when the child is not asked to hate or reject the other beloved parent; that, arguably, is the cruelest thing a parent can do to a child. For when a child comes to hate his Martian father or basil-worshipping mother, he may well come to hate himself also.

Differences between parent and child can be especially salient and conflicted in cases of adoption. For all sorts of reasons, children of adoptions are at higher risks for most all of the problems that distress children and that bring them and their families to treatment. Such was the case with Manuel, a junior high school student who'd been adopted in Guatemala by his single mother. "My mother's a white bitch," he'd complain. "I'm going to kick her fat white ass." Such was the language that Manuel often used to describe his Irish American mother when he was angry. Manuel knew that somewhere in Central America there was a woman who looked like him and whom he looked like. What more poignant metaphor for his sense of not belonging than to contrast his mother's pale white skin with his own dark Guatemalan color? It was easier for Manuel to posit his hurt in a tension that was simplified, that was literally black and white. *Abandonment*—what an overwhelming and near impossible reality for a child or adult to ever make sense of.

Manuel's derision of his mother's whiteness said less about her and more of his own difficulty in valuing himself and his Hispanic heritage, a lack that I worked to fill. When working with children like Manuel, I find it is so important to cherish who they are even when they can't do the same.

How do clinicians convey that? By our good listening and attention to what they bring us. That, above all, tells them they matter to us and the world, through our noticing of their race or culture. I do not hesitate to share with child patients my genuine interest in their culture, which includes my frequent attempts to eat at ethnic restaurants and cook foods from other places. Children are more than happy to help me read a menu that I bring in or to help me research the best way to cook paella. When they bring in or up something about their culture or place of birth, I try to nurture their own revelation and urge them to tell me more, perhaps by drawing me a picture or showing me on a map. Children accurately see our interest in their race or culture as interest in themselves. Should a longer-term patient tell me about a movie or book that relates to who they are, I will attempt to read or watch it. There is no end to the ways that we confirm a child's being and that we ever help him or her to grow more self-accepting and loving too.

As we clinicians work with more people of a certain faith or ethnicity, we learn fast that they are far from all alike. Using rigid assumptions to understand our patients will fail fast and sure. The notion that every Hindi is alike or that their family dynamics are alike is as ridiculous a statement as saying the same about Americans, French people, or Ivy League graduates. We are all simultaneously unique and similar, subject to the same laws of human nature and biology. And yet, while it's pretty obvious that not all Ukrainians or Lutherans are the same, both patients and therapists seem to find some comfort in meeting someone of the same background. This compatibility is to be taken warily. Familiarity can make for an initial ease, and certain cultural sensibilities do carry potential for connection and resonance. But what happens if that is where we stop? The more genuine and open the exploration, the more we will find that someone who looks much like ourselves is in many ways nothing like us at all. To rest too comfortably in our harmony with patients deters us from that candor and progression. Ironically, it can be harder to get to know someone who seems to be just like us.

Over the past years I have treated a young Indian man with Down syndrome, a deaf Hispanic teen, an African American boy with learning disabilities, an autistic Chinese girl, and a Russian child with labile mood. Understanding what these problems can mean within the culture of the home is germane to our work with the children and their families. Consider, for example, all that an adopted immigrant boy from a war-torn country contends with: the trauma of the tragedy he's seen, the loss of his birth family, the stress of moving to a new home in a new land, giving up his mother tongue as he learns English in school and in the community, dealing with dyslexia and childhood asthma, and on and on. Just because an inner-city African American child might bear the effects of prejudice, poverty, crime, and a splintered family doesn't excuse her from having to also grow through and confront all of the other more basic developmental tasks and stresses of childhood. If we think it's hard to manage all of this, we are starting to grasp the burden it puts on the child.

Many years ago I liked to think that I was free of prejudice. When writing a book on children and teachers, I felt quite good as I mailed out the manuscript to an African American professor of education who'd agreed to read it. What a shock when I heard back from him. He took me to task for dozens of comments, like my using the word *darkness* to connote despair or my using the cliché that we might as well have been speaking Chinese. At first, I was irritated and felt that I'd been wrist-slapped by the politically correct police. But what he said slowly sunk in, and when it did, I felt quite bad and quite properly rebuked. That I thought such remarks didn't offend showed my not getting it. It is subtle how our language and sayings and literature regularly betray those biases and stereotypes, even if we don't mean to. It is that prejudicial marinade in which our children love and learn. What does this have to do with your clinical work? Nothing. It has to do with my own clinical work and my learning the hard but necessary way that I, by nature of being different, cannot possibly know what it's like to be African American, Korean, Buddhist, or adopted. Although that professor's critique spurred me to get more sensitive and enlightened, it's greater lesson was the need to recognize and own my inevitable biases and ignorance when it comes to race, culture, and religion.

And that awareness accounts for what may appear to be my greatest omission. I have not spoken as to what it can mean to be a clinician of any other religion, race, or culture. That would be presumptuous and overstepping. More so, it would be a mistake, for I'd have little to add to the generalities I've already proposed. I do know, however, that there is no such thing as a prototypical child therapist of any particular race, color, or religion. I'll leave it to readers to wonder what role, if any, issues of their backgrounds and belief play in their own therapeutic work.

The issues of this chapter deserve so much more, a book of its own. This is but a provocative sampling. And yet, for all of the good books and articles, it is our experience with children and their families and our openness to learn from them that ultimately give us our boot camp and continuing education in understanding and working with people who differ from ourselves. Hour by hour we learn more about who they are, who we are, and what we make as a therapeutic couple. More so, every real person we meet helps us to dismantle any preconceived notions we hold for people as a group or in the hypothetical. They—meaning children and families of any one color or belief—all look alike *only when we can't really see them*.[1]

NOTE

1. If there's any one message I wish to stress in this chapter it is the need, at least for me, to know what I don't know. Nowhere does this seem more important than when considering the issues of race, religion, and culture. I strive to let each new patient teach me who they are, what they believe, what their culture is, and so on. I do, though, recommend one current book that is pragmatic, thorough, and intelligent, edited by experienced therapists knowledgeable on this issue: *Cultural Issues in Play Therapy* (Gil & Drewes, 2005).

17

When Therapy Is Not Enough: Medication

As our scientific understanding of the mind has grown, more attention has focused on developing drugs to treat troubling symptoms and behaviors. Like most advances in science, this explosion of psychotropic medication has both solved and created problems. It has been a godsend to many, while it has harmed some and done not much for the rest. This chapter examines the role of medicine and its implications for children and their therapies.

Often, a primary question when we first meet a child is whether he or she seems to warrant medication. The history that we collect in our evaluation gives us some perspective, though our richest data are from our observations of the child. We ask ourselves whether he is unduly hurting. In assessing him, his and his parents' self-awareness, sensitivity, and sense of drama all need to be taken seriously. Does the child exaggerate her upset, and, if so, for what and whose benefit? There are children, too, who minimize their pain, who've walked around for months or years silently bearing their distress. Do the parents accurately sense their child's ordeal? Do they blow his minor frustrations out of proportion, or, conversely, do they not take his suicidally tinged self-disparaging seriously? Emotional pain is subjective and can't be easily measured as one might check the red blood cell count or test for strep.

Likewise, what do we make of children who exhibit behaviors that cause themselves and others problems and grief but that they claim they cannot control? How do we know what their effort has been? Will our work with them, we wonder, be the key to triggering greater self-control, or do they also need the support of medication? We wallow through the morass, not wanting to either push for unnecessary medication or neglect medical treatment that can bring a child deserved relief and behavioral benefit.

Nine-year-old Toby appeared as depressed as his parents and teacher had described him. He sat perfectly still in his chair and answered my questions with flat and telegraphically short responses. He showed no interest in my toys or me. Toby's parents stressed that, however unmistakably sullen, he never talked of being sad, not liking himself, or wanting to die. "If not for his constant moping about," his mother said with unrecognized irony, "we'd never know anything is wrong with him."

Toby's parents, on the school's suggestion, had hoped that I—despite their knowing that I was a psychologist—might give Toby a prescription for an antidepressant. "We can't stand seeing him like this anymore," his father said.

When I asked Toby himself whether he was as miserable as his parents told me he was, he showed a bit of life. "I hate my parents. I hate myself. And there's nothing anyone or any medicine can do to make me feel any better."

Toby's sudden determination told me much. He had feelings, strong ones. His passivity and gloominess involved unexpressed hostility. Toby was not happy with his life as it was; his proclaiming his helplessness said to me that he wanted help, if only it could be found. His final assertion that no person or drug could help also seemed to ring of some resentment and opposition to his being brought here and to his obvious knowledge of his parents' wish that he be medicated. His parting remark—"You won't tell my parents what I said, will you?"—attested, I thought, to his conflict with and caring for his parents as well as some connecting with me as his potential therapist.

Buoyed by what I saw in Toby and hearing how his parents' frustration stoked their desire that he be medicated, I put off a medical consultation for the time being. "Let's give therapy a go," I suggested, "and we'll give drugs a look at the first sign that they're needed."

They never were.

Why might we delay medication? To begin medication and therapy at the same time can be confusing. If the therapist is not also a psychiatrist, the child must work out new relationships with two clinicians. Most critically, beginning therapy and a new medication together can make for a confounded experiment. If the child shows relief, how do we know whether to credit the medicine or the therapy? Should the child show seeming side effects, how can we be sure they are not born of stress due to a new therapy? While such questions are seldom crystal clear, adding two variables at once may complicate our thinking about the child. In some cases medication can judiciously be stalled to allow the therapy to get going, providing a more solid foundation for drugs should they be needed.

Our slowing down the request for medications can itself be comforting. Parents who've suffered alongside their children for some time may be desperate for help. Our steady welcome and holding, letting them know of our concerned awareness for their child's symptoms, and affirming that we're keeping the question of medication on the front burner can calm their worry. I commonly find child patients just as open to my suggestion that we consider medication more carefully after we've had a chance to get to know each other and to get to see how helpful my work with them might be.

On the other hand, there can be compelling reasons to move ahead with medication early in treatment. We want to ameliorate distress that has already gone on too long or appears of a sort our therapy will not soon reduce. Clinicians may reason, for example, that an antianxiety drug can soften paralyzing panic so as to get the broader treatment off the ground. Because some medicines, such as the popular SSRI antidepressants, require several weeks to reach effective blood levels, clinicians may fear getting another month or two behind the symptom. Clinicians may judge some floridly psychotic or agitated children to need quick biological help to regroup and become accessible to life and intervention. Rather than conflict with the play and talk we do, mollifying these distressing conditions can enable some child patients to better tolerate and cooperate with the therapy.

As one who has neither the legal privilege nor the expertise to prescribe, I trust the psychiatrists and psychopharmacologists I consult to help me figure things out. Their experience often knows how to better decipher, for instance, the level, depth, and treatability of a child's depression. As these prescribing clinicians inevitably have overwrought schedules, I often encourage new patients to make an appointment now (which will be many weeks or even months in the future). I urge the parent not to pressure prescribing clinicians but to comply with the pace of their assessment. In my experience, child psychiatrists are just as cautious not to prescribe when it's either unnecessary or not so clear. I routinely see child patients walk out of their medication evaluations without a prescription. But even in cases where my child patients end up not using drugs, my and their consulting with psychiatry has proved consoling, insightful, and facilitating of therapeutic progress.

The child who is referred because of impulsivity, distractibility, hyperactivity, and misbehavior presents a slightly different problem. The job of teasing out depression, worry, neurological issues, and environment from inattention can be tedious and time consuming. Such children typically have neither an interest in nor a tolerance for discussing their feelings; they often have no wish for therapy. These children, particularly if they have had less-than-successful trials of treatment previously, also may be clearer candidates for medication. I have tended to err in the opposite direction, being too conservative in terms of medication, waiting too long to recommend drugs that can help a distracted child learn better or be less frenetic. Because medication can be a catalyzing factor in therapy with these children, it might well be initiated sooner rather than later in a treatment.

When a therapy proceeds well enough to support its continuing but fails to bring needed relief soon enough and nothing in the process leads us to believe that great improvement is just around the corner, it also may be time to obtain a pharmacological consultation. Before calling for an evaluation, however, we may benefit by discussing the matter with the child for whom medication is being considered. Talking with children about the severity of their distress, the frustration of their distractibility, and the depths of their pessimism lays the groundwork to explore the possibility of medical intervention.

Care must be taken here to put the notion of medicine into the context of the therapy. A simplistic "therapy isn't working, so we better try drugs" will likely make the child feel a failure and exacerbate whatever distress exists. In fact, if a question remains about whether the therapy or we as therapists are helping that child, we need to broach that topic first and separately. A child should not be given medicine to avert our own frustration over a lack of clinical progress or understanding, though consulting with a child psychiatrist or psychopharmacologist may show that we've overlooked something beneficial.

Some children are readily open to medicine. They welcome the possibility of a life that looks less dark or feels less panicked. Some children are ambivalent, wondering if a drug can really help and wary of its side effects or potential for addiction. Others, sometimes those most needing it, are vehemently opposed, phobically fearing that it might poison them or change their personalities. Hypervigilant to any intrusion into their body or mind, they see drugs as devil stuff meant to control them as the mistrusted authorities in their world see fit. I've seen more than a few children who suffer horrendous self-hatred feel themselves undeserving of a medicine that might lift their guilt and depression and maybe make them happier.

Taking a week or two (or many more) to help a child work through his feelings about medication is usually time well spent. A child or family who holds a cooperative attitude toward medication will provide the consulting psychiatrist with the most reliable and useful data, resulting in the best-informed prescription and optimum compliance. A child who is dragged to the psychiatrist, sometimes unavoidably, will be apt to fight the interview as well as resist the medicine. As a rule, whatever useful exploring a child does around the issue of medication holds more generalizable value for his therapy and self-examination as a whole.

It is ideal when we can refer to psychiatrists with whom we can communicate and who have an understanding for the kind of therapy we do. Most psychiatrists, however busy, appreciate the therapist's observations with reference to the child's symptoms, function, response to the therapeutic relationship, and feelings toward medication. Their job—assessing and prescribing for dozens of children whom they see for limited periods of time—gets tougher every day, making them ever more amenable to whatever information or thoughts we can offer. Although they tend to know the medicines best, we've had the luxury of knowing our patients in ways they cannot. It's always fascinating, too, to hear of the material the consulting psychiatrist often garners when meeting our patients, revelations (particularly about symptoms) that have somehow passed under our eyes or over our heads or that the child chose not to share with us. And, of course, the many psychiatrists who also do therapy are in the unique position of seeing both sides. While this dual role implies potential blind spots, it also can allow for a powerful, highly responsive, and well-integrated treatment within a relationship with one provider.

In the course of deeper and more tumultuous therapies, it is not rare for the child to undergo anguished phases where troubling behaviors or unsettling symptoms reappear with a fury. These therapeutic crises can scare the child, her parents, and the therapist, discouraging everyone along the way. The utmost care needs to be taken to assess what's transpiring. Rushing to medication risks undermining the hard work that is progressing and giving children the impression that their darkest and ugliest innards cannot be borne by those they depend on (their parents, their therapist). Confused and thrown as these therapeutic upheavals can make us, the child needs us to hold tight, to resist such pressures as the fear of legal repercussions, public opinion, and school disapproval that can propel us toward unnecessary action that may sabotage the therapy and waste the therapeutic opportunity of the crisis.

> Twelve-year-old Steven was a nervous wreck. His rigid body resembled a robot's, and his tense face showed only dread. He'd been referred for high anxiety, obsessions of being harmed, a compulsive need to wash his hands and play with numbers, and constant frustration. Apprehensive of infectious disease and the dangers of intimacy, he'd withdrawn from peers and could barely function in the child- and germ-filled atmosphere of the school.
>
> Steven made great progress during the first year of treatment. Over countless sessions full of primitive explosions, shame, and repentance, Steven grew much more accepting of his enraged jealousy of a deaf brother who got most of his parents' attention. Although he stopped doting on his brother, the boys grew closer and more compatible. His compulsions all but disappeared, and he became an engaged, if a bit shy, member of the sixth-grade culture.
>
> These wondrous gains made his sudden disintegration that much more disconcerting. Within a week's time Steven appeared to lose all his hard-won progress. He refused to eat, fearing his food was tainted by his mother's hands. Cruelty absolutely ruled his treatment of his brother, leading Steven, a bright boy, to learn curses and other phrases

in sign language to put his brother down. He entirely withdrew in school, breaking down to crying jags that required his leaving class. Most disturbing of all, he took to punching his own head and twisting his fingers so hard he'd bruise his own knuckles. I learned all of this on one morning via frantic calls from the school principal, his guidance counselor, his parents, and even Steven himself, who asked to see me a day early.

In that hour Steven could do no more than cry and repeatedly say that he had no idea what was happening to him. "Maybe I'm going crazy," was all he could come up with. For several weeks I received frantic calls from school and home, at first encouraging me to get Steven some medication, eventually questioning what I was doing with the boy.

Fending off my own self-doubt, I reread session notes and thought hard about all that had happened over the past 13 months. I worried about his disintegrating. "Should I be taking swifter action?" I kept asking myself. Yet I was certain there was some good reason for this regression and feared doing anything that might throw a wrench into what might be a therapeutic opening as much as it was a challenge.

It wasn't until the third week of doubled sessions that we hit pay dirt. Passing my children's bicycles in the driveway, Steven remembered dreaming that his brother had been run down by a train. "He was riding like mad to catch up with me. He didn't hear the train or the signal." Steven began to punch the chair.

"He didn't really die," I said.

"But," Steven said, his chest heaving with emotion, his fists whacking the side of his head. "I wanted him to." Steven punched himself again. "I wanted him to die." Steven fell to the floor, wailing.

Late in the hour, relieved of his enormous hurt, Steven figured out that his dream had come the day after he'd tried to ditch his brother at the mall. Immediately feeling guilty, he'd raced back to get his brother, only to see him running wildly through the mall looking for Steven. "He tripped over a trash can he was so upset," Steven recalled with a half cry, half laugh.

Although he required a good several weeks more of therapy to get back to where he'd been, Steven soon was growing even more quickly than before. We'd stayed the course together.

There are times, conversely, where child patients are reexperiencing a trauma or loss that it's clear will not resolve itself quickly. Although therapy is frequently arduous and painful and despite the teachings as to religious salvation, inordinate suffering is neither a virtue nor necessarily healthful. A child's hurt, while often accompanying the working through of bad experiences and coming to terms with his limitations, need not be intolerable for growth and repair to proceed. In such cases I have referred my patients for short to moderate courses of medication to keep their distress to bearable levels. In none of the cases has the medication instantly made the child happy and carefree. The drugs dulled the crippling anxieties and depression that have been tormenting a child beyond belief, enabling the therapeutic work to continue unabated.

While psychotropic medications have their place, some skepticism is warranted. Many medications have significant side effects. Some of these, such as the potential damage to the heart or pancreas, require parents to make difficult decisions. I've seen parents tortured over this choice: watching their child's pain and worried that their decision to okay a medicine will cause real physical harm. We've learned the hard way that sometimes no reported side effects means no side effects thus far.

Therapists can help the child and family monitor as well as manage less life-threatening side effects. Highly suggestive or sensitive children often do best by not knowing all of the various adverse effects their medication can elicit. Ample discussion of the child's feelings about taking medicine—our job even more than that of the prescriber—can help to minimize untoward reactions. We also can help to confirm or assuage parents' anxieties about side effects they are unsure they are seeing, supporting contact with the child's psychiatrist when necessary. When we see that something is not quite right—strange motorisms with an antipsychotic—we can make sure that the prescribing clinician is notified.

Not only can premature or frivolous medicating interfere with treatment, but drugs that overly numb a child or cloud or slow her thinking can obstruct her functioning outside and inside therapy. I have seen Ritalin help many, but I've also seen it exacerbate underlying anxieties, causing obsessive children to obsess more. This rigidifying effect on feeling and thinking, besides feeling uncomfortable and strange, can deenergize a therapy, making children much less accessible to themselves and the freer aspects of self-exploration. Just as often, though, alleviating an overwhelming symptom does not defuse a child's motivation to do the hard work of therapy. Aptly administered drugs—antidepressants, for example—can do precisely the opposite, mobilizing a child who otherwise lacks the energy or hopefulness to engage in a treatment.

Particularly with the diagnosis of attention-deficit hyperactivity disorder (ADHD), children need to understand the meaning of their taking drugs. Some are prone to interpret it as a straitjacket in tablet form. Parents, teachers, and therapists quick to attribute a good day to medicine or a bad day to its absence can unwittingly promote a child's abdication of personal responsibility. The drug is intended to help children organize and attend so they can have good experiences and feel successful. However, children often come to see the power that the adults in their lives attribute to that little pill. Ongoing discussion will monitor the child's feeling about the medicine and its effects, with the goal of raising the child's awareness of the effects of his own behavior and self-control.

Another major jeopardy of medication is that it can detour necessary or better intervention. Hopeful that a pill can fix their child's hurts and misbehavior (and who can blame them?), some parents are prone to shelve the more plodding work of therapy temporarily while they wait for an appointment at an ADHD clinic, for example, or for an antidepressant to reach therapeutic blood levels. Just as some prefer psychological explanations, others would rather hear that their child's difficulties are purely neurological or congenital and have little to do with anything that has gone on at the home. Therapists can counter this risk by supporting parents' interest in medication and robustly acknowledging the temperamental and biological bases of our beings, all the while promoting the need to continue nonmedical efforts to improve the child's environment.

Regardless of how hard we work and how skilled the prescribing clinicians, there will be many cases that do not flourish. Psychotic and enraged children may need drug trial after drug trial, no one medication helping for more than a limited time. Children and parents may work for months to grow comfortable with the idea of medication, only to discover that it brings no miracles. And, as we all know, there are parents who won't consider medication under any circumstances, however awful their child's problems and internal life.

Drugs deserve their rightful and major place in the treatment of children. When prescribed wisely and introduced thoughtfully into a child's therapy, they can enormously facilitate a child's relief, functioning, and therapeutic growth. Administered carelessly or against a child's will, they can be useless or worse. Attending to the meanings that medication holds for children, their parents, and their treatment can have everything to do with enhancing the drug therapy, the play and talk therapy, and their joint success.

18

I Can Name That Tune in Six Sessions: Managed Care and Evidence-Based Treatment

Although Bob Dylan had bigger things in mind, he was right that the times have been a-changing. And nowhere have those changes been more apparent and pressing than in the field of child mental health. Witness the creation and explosion of health maintenance organizations (HMOs) and managed care, the shrinking of insurance benefits, and a societal mind-set that wants everything to be fast and drive-through. This penultimate chapter will discuss the current landscape in hopes of helping child therapists tease and flesh out their own clinical attitudes, methods, and ethics. I begin by describing the controversy and tensions that exist, followed by more pragmatic ways to adapt the old and new ways.

As you know, I come from a psychodynamic orientation. Although the theories and techniques of the psychodynamic are distinguishable from the Rogerian or child-centered perspective, they are highly compatible. We both honor relationships, inner worlds, feelings, family, and a drive toward health, and we both see acceptance, respectfulness, trust, empathy, good listening and communication, patience, and the like as therapeutic requisites. Although child-centered therapists, like Virginia Axline and Clark Moustakas, might not use exactly the same language or concepts to describe what they do, a large number of child therapists and counselors employ some kind of experience-informed amalgam of our two approaches. After all, those who study and are open to human experience and relations—whether a novelist or a child therapist—often come to approximately equal truths and insights that guide their work and world view. And so, being unabashedly of this therapeutic ilk and perspective, I can only begin to make sense of evidence-based treatments through that existing lens and sensibility. Having many years of experience conducting longer-term relationship-based therapy and seeing the profound benefits they've wrought, I am admittedly a stubborn customer. The evidence-based researchers want to see proof of an intervention's worth. Well, in a comparable way, even if not fitting their more scientific bent, I need to see proof to steer me away from the data I've collected hour after hour from patients, supervisors, and colleagues for more than a quarter of a century.

What stokes my skepticism of the new therapies? Foremost, the patients I meet take a good deal of time to feel safe, forge an alliance, and open up before moving on to face reality, confront their problems, and change. When as a younger clinician I'd first heard presentations on short-term treatments, my initial reaction was to simultaneously chuckle and marvel. The patients I heard about were accomplishing great things in a handful of meetings. I could only imagine how much healthier these people were than I was. Were these clinicians treating the same patients whom I treated? Were they seeking the same growth and relief? Were my therapeutic aims larger and broader, or, I had to ask, were those therapists able to do more and do faster with their new techniques and skills?

I also have theoretical reservations. Although I'd minored in neurobiology and hold great appreciation for our biological destiny, I know that other things matter. While everything is biologically based—every feeling, fear, memory, and idea is formed, stored, and conducted through the physical world of the nervous system—it is also psychologically experienced. For a child to be human is to continually find and make meaning out of what she, her body and mind, experiences. Yet I cannot find any recognition of that in these new treatments. Nor is there any mention of empathy and feeling understood, touchstones of human connection. Psychological conflict and the ways that children's psyches naturally protect themselves from these hurts are missing, as are guilt, shame, and regret, all-important and often pervasive powers in a child's and parent's life. Over the years, adherents of the psychoanalytic school have rightly taken it on the chin for emphasizing the individual and internal while neglecting the influences of family, peers, society, culture, race, religion, socioeconomic status, and environment. But I seldom have found these factors in the theories or strategies of evidence-based treatments.

I acknowledge that the new empiricists have plenty of faults to find with psychodynamic therapy. We have little science and few verifiable studies to defend our brand of therapy. And that isn't their fault. To those critics, our terminology and concepts appear fantastic and irreducible. We see what we want to see, so they judge, even if what we see are the emperor's new (invisible and nonexistent) clothes. Over the years, wrong turns and abuses of the old school have not aided our cause. Bettelheim cruelly blamed so-called refrigerator mothers for causing their children's autism. Many old-time psychoanalysts practiced a stern withholding and patriarchal form of therapy that left many patients, especially women, without help or worse and that often blamed them for their hurts and trauma, though, of course, the sins of our forefathers do not make us sinners any more than do the shortcomings and mistakes of the empirical therapists negate the good deeds of their clinical descendants. They call us on the carpet for taking too long to do our therapy and, by way of our having no objectified measures and concepts, for having no easy-to-see and validated markers to guide the work, assess its progress (or lack thereof), and determine when it's complete. The explanations we put forth leave them untouched and impressed mostly by our wild clinical imaginations.

Just as the evidence-based researchers question our methods and madness, it would be easy to return the favor. Why, I wonder, do evidence-based researchers often discount what patients say and care about? High-functioning autistic authors, for example, write with indignation about their sense that the autism experts seem to think they know more about them than they do themselves, noting how seldom, if ever, they are questioned as to what they think and feel (Baggs, 2000; Hall, 2000). Evidence-based workers frequently rebuke psychodynamic clinicians for not heeding the research, for blindly following their unproven techniques. Paradoxically, if anecdotally, I have found just the opposite. Most psychodynamic therapists I know keep abreast of and employ biological, behavioral, educational, and other methods. More behavioral and focused clinicians believe they understand psychodynamic theory, data, and clinical work well enough to critique it, but they often know little more than stereotypical headlines, as if what we do all day is to interpret penises and vaginas to children lying prone on mahogany and velvet fainting couches. Learning and mastering psychodynamic understanding and applying it is no small feat.

These empiricists also do not seem much interested in the new science that corroborates psychodynamic principles. The hard findings of neuroscience are increasingly supporting analytic concepts such as repression, defenses, and the unconscious. An intriguing recent study from the burgeoning field of social neuroscience, for instance, has found tangible physiological evidence for the mysteriously resonant and empathic communication that psychodynamic therapists know and live by daily. Many other scientific studies are uncovering hard data that synchronize with psychodynamic conceptualizations concerning attachment, separation, and the mechanisms of therapy. Rather than analytic propaganda, this nascent field of study is being advanced and supported by legitimate and prominent researchers in neurology, psychiatry, and neuroscience. In a lovely paradox, "neuroscience, the very discipline that kicked Freud off his pedestal in the last few decades of the 20th century, may eventually return his brainchild, the talking cure, to prominence in the 21st" (Kendall, 2003). More recent outcome studies are also showing evidence for the sometimes superior merit of talking therapies, which harkens us to admit that the evidence-based researchers are correct. We should be doing studies to testify to the benefits we know our relationship-based approaches can bring.

As a primarily psychodynamic therapist who integrates and considers other approaches, I recognize the merit of evidence-based research to child treatment. Who can argue against the search for more timely, cost-effective, and readily transferable interventions for helping children and their families, not just in America but throughout the world? There is no virtue in prolonging a child's suffering or difficulties one more hour than is necessary; we all wish to alleviate it as fast as we can. While I value the kind of work I do, I can't believe it fits every child of every circumstance everywhere. Yet what I fear and what fuels my obvious defensiveness is the sweeping aspect of the evidence-based research protocol. It is as dangerous as it's mistaken to entrust any single clinical orientation as the gatekeeper of therapeutic truth. We live in an imperfect world that overflows with enough pain and dysfunction for all of us to work on reducing and preventing.

But we are child therapists—I'm speaking for myself now—and come Monday morning, we must climb off our soapbox and work with the children and families who need us. What are we to do as we struggle to practice against this backdrop and under the constraints that today's health care place on us? In general and as glib as it sounds, the place to begin is with the child. What in the ideal, we ask ourselves, does this child need therapeutically? Once we have some idea, then we rein it in and adapt it to available resources (i.e., time, money, therapeutic goals). To compromise before we've assessed and conceptualized the child's troubles can risk our short-circuiting valuable observation, interacting, and problem solving. To realize that the child who an HMO has allotted six weeks of therapy really needs many months worth can be preferable to blindly persuading ourselves that six sessions are all the child needs. Reducing cognitive dissonance may be good for the therapist's stress level but can distract him from the reality of what actually exists and is warranted. Appreciating the complexity and depth of what we deal with can inform and transform what we make of our much more limited time with the child.

I know many therapists who strive to adapt much of what they do in longer therapies to the short term. They create trust, listen with empathy, and heed what the child thinks and feels while also attempting to motivate the family's awareness of what they can do to help. Even as these therapists out of necessity utilize more directive and proactive strategies, they do so within nurturing and therapeutic relationships. They carve out, at least in their heads, what they can achieve reasonably while being up front as to what they cannot attain. These child clinicians creatively search for and summon alternative resources to support and compensate for what they won't have the luxury to accomplish in the therapy proper.

PLAYING TO ORDER

Let's get practical. Let's address specific symptoms, issues, and situations for which children are referred for treatment. Taking each problem one by one, we will ask, How can a child therapist responsibly adapt their relationship-based treatment, psychodynamic or child centered, to contemporary practice? The impressive study of John Weisz (2004) will serve as our guide to the current state of evidence-based treatment for children. I refer all child therapists to this book as a thoughtful, thorough, and provocative entry to both evidence-based treatment research and its findings.

Please note that the following discussion attempts to integrate psychodynamic with evidence-based treatments. We will not address biological psychiatry and medication here.

Simple Fears

Evidence-based treatment research (EBTR) found four methods to be effective with simple phobias of children: modeling (watching another child not be fearful), systematic desensitization, graduated exposure, and self-talk (cognitive-behavioral). These methods all worked well and fairly quickly. In retrospect, it's likely that my similar success in working with simple fears is attributable to my employing aspects of these well-defined interventions. For example, I quickly and with gentle firmness urge children to work their way up to facing their fear behaviorally. I teach them how to counter their negative thinking, replacing it with their own or my voice cheering them onward. And I show them techniques to relax and meditate as a way to reduce their anxiety. I am sure that behavioral researchers would see and identify themselves in the efficacy of my therapy for simple fears. Given how common such fears are, it behooves psychodynamic and child-centered therapists to learn these techniques and to follow the research as their methods grow more refined and incisive.

Anxiety Disorders

EBTR identified a cognitive-behavioral method (called the Coping Cat Program) as effective for generalized anxiety, separation anxiety, and social phobia. Again, these are common disorders in the child therapy office. We should learn what we can about this type of treatment. I regularly employ self-talk, cognitive restructuring, parent management, testing of faulty beliefs, and other aspects of this method within my broader therapeutic relationship. Because anxieties and phobias are often much more complex and woven with other issues, including inner fantasies and conflicts, I find that combining the crucial methods of the cognitive-behavioral within the psychodynamic relationship makes for a powerfully restorative intervention. I must add that in certain neurotic children, merely talking and playing in an accepting and empathic environment can alleviate their level of anxiety and also make them more resilient to the anxiety that life inevitably entails. And, of course, group therapy can sometimes be beneficial to the socially phobic child.

Depression

As with anxiety, EBTR found that cognitive-behavioral treatment works well with childhood depression. Newer studies with adults suggest that the psychodynamic variety of talking therapy works also. Again, I routinely ask depressed children to self-talk and question their negative thinking, just as I integrate affective education and other elements of cognitive-behavioral technique. However, the psychodynamic relationship brings the greater benefit of creating a space in which the child can grow to endure, bear, shed, understand, and overcome their hurt. While I believe that we are all born with certain liabilities—such as the propensity under stress for anxiety, depression, skin rashes, stomachaches, and so on—in my considerable clinical experience I've seen few childhood depressions that don't involve a lot of personal meaning, meaning to be respected, examined, and deciphered for the child's benefit. For example, it is well established that young children of depressed mothers are at risk for depression and other symptoms. Such children often and ably use play and talk to express their frustration and hurt and to find a place and person (the therapist) who possesses the innate enthusiasm, optimism, energy, and self-love to enjoy being with the child and who can help the child rediscover her own joy and vitality. In my view, cognitive-behavioral treatments are limited in how much of that sadness it can lighten and how much of the child's spontaneity it can ignite.

Conduct Disorders

This is a complicated group. For the sociopathic teenager who truly lacks a conscience, talking therapy is too little too late. Research suggests that even boot camp and tough-love interventions may not be enough. For the delinquent child who is on the fence—who lacks some conscience and self-control but who has at least some kernel of caring, humanity, and wish to do better—a relationship with someone who believes in his goodness itself can be a powerful buoy to slow down and maybe reverse his descent. EBTR-proven treatments include anger management, behavioral parent guidance, parent–child interaction therapy, and problem-solving skills treatment. Given the unfortunate frequency with which such children are referred, all child therapists should be skilled in these treatments or should refer the children to clinicians who are skilled. In many cases, parents bring such children late to treatment, usually as teenagers, adding the extra burden for therapists to get moving as quickly as possible. Child therapists cannot afford to lose or waste another year or two of impotent treatment. When it comes to issues of conscience, crime, violence, and the like, therapists sadly face a race with time in the hope that they can steady a teenager before he does more damage to himself or removes himself from society and the privilege of outpatient therapy.

Attentional Disorders

Children with problems of attention are an infinitely varied group. Fortunately, there is good research that ever works to tease out the many species of attention-deficit hyperactivity disorder (ADHD) from one another. For sure, some such children have a neurological difference that stimulants help immediately. EBTR found that behavioral training, teaching parents how to manage these children, was effective. When meeting these children, child therapists frequently use their entire toolbox of strategies. Attention deficits, can reflect, as examples, disorganizing anxiety, learning issues, social phobia, preoccupation, excessive daydreaming that fends off narcissistic injury and low self-esteem, distress of an abusive home or one in which parents fight, obsessive thinking, and hypervigilance secondary to trauma, hunger, and neglect. How do we treat these varied forms of ADHD? With everything we've got—the psychodynamic as well as the behavioral and psychopharmacological. And yes, we all agree on the relevance and value of parent guidance (i.e., behavioral management training) to such parents.

After addressing simple fears, anxiety, depression, conduct, and attentional disorders, we have pretty much run out of EBTR-proven interventions.

What does that leave? An enormous number of the children who come daily to clinics and private therapy offices. And those are the populations, in my view, that most need the help that psychodynamic (and client-centered) child therapy can give. Consider the length and breadth of this list and reflect on your own clients and patients.

The Borderline or Bipolar Child

Call these children, usually boys, whatever you wish—bipolar, border-line, oppositional, and so on. Clinicians have been seeing these children longer than I have been a psychologist. In my experience, they are a mixed group. Some have horrid home lives and trauma, others seem to have been born with exquisitely fragile esteems and labile moods. What works? No quick fix, that's for sure. I've had good success with an intensive therapy that pays a lot of attention to what the child feels and the seemingly minute stresses—the insults and trials, the slights and arrows with which they perpetually feel assaulted—helping them to rec-ognize and process their intense and impulsive reactions. Concepts such as overly harsh consciences, unrelenting pursuit of perfection, and over-whelming shame spotlight our work and clarify our understanding of the misery and self-loathing that pervades their daily existence. It involves ego strengthening, empathic failures and their repair, emotional educa-tion, and a lot of grieving. As you can guess, teaching parents how to manage such children is also critical. Parents of such children tend to feel helpless and defeated. They are also prone to oscillate between the unhealthy extremes of overindulgence and punitive punishment (both are ineffective). Teaching them how to set firm and reliable limits in a loving and nurturing context has been a central piece of my work with these families.

Asperger's and High-Functioning Autism

For years I have practiced and written about the worth of traditional, if modified, talk-and-play therapy with high-functioning autistic and Asperger children. The field of autism has been prejudiced against such a possibility. Out of more than 2,000 articles the leading journal of autism has published, not one has dealt with playing or talking therapy with such children. I am convinced that no rigidly ordained treatment will ever be shown to be the most effective therapy for these wonderful and surprisingly rich children. Play therapy should be adjunct to other critical interventions involving education, language therapy, social groups and training, and parent guidance.

Learning Disabilities

Traditional therapy does a good job of helping a child realize, accept, and cope with a learning issue. Children cannot compensate and master a deficit until they have owned it, until they have admitted to themselves that they have a condition for which they need help. Overcoming the narcissistic injury of having a learning problem is arduous yet can permit a child to become a gracious and constructive help taker, self-checker, and compensatory learner.

Suicidality

Nothing can help a child or teen deal with suicidal impulses more than can the profound holding of a therapeutic relationship. Children who try to kill themselves are desperate and cannot see a way out, even when a door to a brighter place may be mere inches away. Dragnet-inspired third degrees by clinicians running down a laundry list of questions to ask a suicidal teen does little to make a child want to stay alive. But being listened to, taken seriously, empathized with, and promised hope can help a child choose life. Sharing dark and ugly thoughts with a caring and steady therapist can immediately lift one's spirit and make one feel less alone and alien with that hurt and fear. Engaging the suicidal child in his desperate state can energize and help to jump-start the therapeutic relationship, motivate the child to work at unraveling his wish to die, and restore his will to live.

Attachment Disorders

How can a short-term, behavioral treatment ever replace a caring, deep, engaged, empathic, responsive, trustworthy [fill in the blank] relationship for a child with a true attachment disorder? Yes, psychodynamic therapy takes time, but it is the shortest and quickest route toward real attachment.

Trauma

Not so clear. Traditional talking therapy can help a great deal. But so can short-term models involving more structured interventions (e.g., programmed grief work), support groups, and other ancillary resources.

Schizoid and Selective Mutism

I am not equating these problems. Again, in my experience it is a steady and patient relationship that ultimately can draw these children outward.

Down Syndrome

I have had very good experience in conducting traditional psychotherapy with such children. We often forget that such children must deal with all of the developmental and psychological tasks all children undergo in addition to the formidable stresses and hurts that their being different and limited implies. I have also seen them benefit from more structured cognitive and behavioral treatments or those that involve planned activities, social interaction, and group treatment. The children and teens with Down syndrome who I've met are, on the average, a very open, emotionally available, and motivated population that makes good use of most any resource offered to them.

Adjustment Disorders and Life Problems

Talking with a good and therapeutic listener can work miracles with a child experiencing some transient stress, such as a family tragedy or loss, parent separation or divorce, or family illness. With relatively healthy and accessible children and teenagers, group treatments, support groups, and structured short-term programs (both community and school based) can also bring relief and enable children to move on.

To close this section, I need to stress that, while it can feel to psychodynamic clinicians as if evidence-based research is hostile to the children and therapy we work with, it is not. I know that the leaders of the child evidence-based movement, such as John Weisz and Alan Kazdin, would run to bless our approach to therapy if they read studies that proved it to them. For example, in Weisz's (2004) massive and admirable meta-analysis of more than 1,500 child therapy outcome studies, he applied the same rigor and dismissal to all sorts of cognitive, behavioral, and gimmick-laden interventions. His study was not out to get us; it was out to get inadequate outcome research and to find proven methods. But, as he concludes, the foremost issue for future evidence-based research is the need to "build evidence-based treatments for a broadened array of problems and disorders" (p. 449). It is here—with the messy, complex, and deep problems of children and families—that psychodynamic child therapy will sustain and shine, for it is there that we ever prove the mettle and powers of our therapy. The fact that it costs time and money is undeniably an economic consideration for both families and society. But that hard reality does not itself discount either its value or its lessons.[1]

NOTE

1. I have relied on Dr. Weisz's latest review (2004) on evidence-based treatments to accurately represent the current state of knowledge. Clinicians are urged to learn more about his Network on Youth Mental Care, a large-scale evidence-based treatment research program. Readers might wish to see the analyst Doris Silverman's (2006) discussion on the relation and challenge of evidence-based practice to the psychoanalytic field. And, as *brief treatment* is yet one more clinical topic on which I lack expertise, I'll nonetheless mention a smattering of brief treatment models to give an idea of how far they can range and how much they can differ: Corwin's (2001) narrative constructivist models, Sifneos's (2004) short-term anxiety-provoking model, Basch's (1995) psychodynamic brief treatment, and Selekman's (2002) brief treatment model for adolescents—though I need to add that being brief or short term does not necessarily equal being effective or evidence proven.

19

All's Well That Ends Well: Closing Therapy

All good things must come to an end, and that is just as true for therapy. Termination can follow a brief treatment or one that traverses much of a child's childhood. Planned or spontaneous, willing or forced, smooth or tumultuous, discouraging or encouraging, for good reason or bad, satisfying or much less so, termination can take many forms. This final chapter examines the simultaneously universal and varied ways in which children (and their parents) leave therapy as well as the equally common and diverse ways that we, their therapists, help or hinder their doing so.

To begin our look at endings and before addressing the optimal criteria for proper endings, we must recognize that many therapies end for other than clinically good reasons.

Owen's therapy had been having a positive effect. His violent temper and rabid defiance toward authority were both quieting. Even his mother, a most critical woman who'd put me through the third degree before letting me near her son, was looking pleased. But my refusal to shut her divorced husband out of Owen's therapy (and, as she tried, out of the boy's life) led her to end therapy abruptly and with no notice. Only at my insistence did she grudgingly give the boy and me a dozen or so minutes to say good-bye, a good-bye that consisted mostly of my confirming his dazed disbelief at his mother's unreasonableness. "This is awful," I said softly, with a minute left. Owen shook his head in sad agreement. "You can call me or write anytime," I added, doubting that he ever would. Owen left with his mother, knowing, it seemed, that he would never again see me.

In any suddenly aborted treatment, we do our best to acknowledge the traumatic ending, the value of our relationship, and the work that has been done and offer any wisdom or strategies that might help the child cope without us. This applies, for example, to treatments that are increasingly being shut down by insurance companies or health maintenance organizations no longer willing to pay for them.

Felicia was a sweet child who'd put her dozen or so sessions to good use. Her palpable anxiety and school phobia had diminished, though she remained exquisitely vulnerable to the stresses of school and daily life. Having informed me that their insurance company's benefits had changed, allotting us one more session, her parents made clear that, even with the modest reduced fee I immediately offered, her therapy would be ending. "She's much better," they said. "We haven't gotten a call to pick her up from school in almost two months."

Wondering what other resistance played a role here, I tried my best to hear the parents' misgivings, hoping to incite their own judgment that, however well Felicia and her therapy had been doing, she needed more. Although I wanted to tell them all the bad things that might happen if Felicia was to quit, to frighten them into staying, I refrained. I knew that they could worry at least as well as I about their daughter's future. Moreover, sensing there was a likelihood that these parents were going to go off with Felicia, the last thing I wished to do was hang swords of doom over their heads to further strain their already stressed life.

Once it was apparent that they had made up their minds, I bargained for one additional session, making them an offer (of a fee) they couldn't refuse. Having thus doubled the number of ending sessions available, I used one with Felicia, to close up her work with me.

I devoted the all-important second one to her parents, to provide them some strategies to help Felicia cope without therapy as well as to have a bit more time to cultivate our alliance in hopes of further nurturing their nurturing of Felicia; I sought also to bid them adieu with as much connection and good feeling as possible so they would not be shy to return to me or another therapist should their daughter need help.

Tragically, I have twice seen parents close down their child's therapy because it was helping. In both cases a child was hated by her dutiful mother. Although the children had made great internal gains in their work with me, the weight of their mothers' unwavering and unquestioned dislike for them proved too much. The little time I had to end treatment with each child was spent in sad farewell, reminding her of her self-worth, ways in which I'd miss her, and, most important, ways to continue fending off her mother's hatred and to keep open to the good love that she, the child deserved and that I know others would give her.

Parents aren't the only ones to stop ongoing therapies in their tracks. The therapist in training or who is changing jobs frequently brings good therapies to an end well before their time.

"You're full of shit." During his yearlong therapy, Quentin had occasionally cursed in passing frustration, but he'd never aimed his swears at me. The 12-year-old looked down as he rolled a small toy car back and forth on my desk.

"What's the matter?" I asked, knowing that it was our terminating, but lost as to his accusation.

"I thought I could trust you."

He'd felt lied to or betrayed, I understood. But about what? Our ending? I'd given him fair warning at the start of our work that, as an intern, I'd be leaving the training site and his therapy come the last week of June (and that week was almost here). I knew he hadn't forgotten because he'd interrupted me to mention it when I first broke the news that we had only eight weeks of therapy left.

"Everyone else lies to me, but I thought you were different." Quentin's voice cracked with disappointment and hurt. There was no joke or showboating here.

Had I neglected to bring something I'd said I would? I didn't think so, but anything was possible.

"You act so sad about leaving me." Quentin continued, in a mockingly saccharine voice. "We worked so hard together." "I wish we didn't have to stop." "We only have eight weeks left."

"Those are my words," I said, impressed by the clarity of Quentin's listening and remembering.

"What bullshit," Quentin again accused. "Is someone putting a gun to your head?"

I tilted my head, unsure what he was asking.

"Is someone making you leave this building at gunpoint?" he asked.

"No."

"Is someone making you take that new job?"

I shook my head no.

"You'll be making more money there?"

I nodded that I would be.

"But you don't really want that job?" Quentin had dropped the car and was now walking about the office with the swagger of a prosecuting attorney, confident in his rightness. "You'd *really* rather stay here forever, making less money working with me? Isn't that right?"

I was at a loss for words. Quickly getting his message, I wanted to right the wrong I'd done. I wanted to answer honestly. But I didn't want to hurt his feelings. And besides, the answer wasn't that black and white. Yes, I wanted the new job, but I also would have liked to keep working with Quentin. But this boy—who in his confronting of me was showing me so much of the gains he'd made over the past year—rescued me with yet another question.

"Why couldn't you just say the truth? Quentin," he said, becoming me, "we've done a lot of good work together, and I'm going to miss you. But I've found a new job that I'm very excited about. I'll be making more money and will get to be the boss. Why couldn't you just say that?" Quentin asked. "D'you think I'm too weak to take it? Do you think lying made me feel better?" His voice grew louder. "Do you think after all this time I wouldn't be happy for you? Do you? Do you?" Quentin began to cry. "Fuck, isn't that what friends are for?"

Feeling ashamed, a loser, a clinical has-been that never was, I could barely face Quentin. Everything he said was true. I hadn't shown him any of the relief and pride I felt to be completing my internship and graduate training. I hadn't shown any of the pride and pleasure I felt anticipating a real job for which I'd be paid more than a pittance. Denying those truths had cast doubt over the truths I did express: my true sadness about leaving Quentin and my wish that we were just embarking on a therapy to last years and years. Quentin understandably didn't know what to believe.

To make matters worse, by suggesting that everyone but me was ending his therapy—that it was mandated by the rules of the hospital, the requirements of my graduate program, the demands of the new clinic—I conveniently excused myself of all responsibility for leaving Quentin. In fact, the way I'd put it to him, I wasn't leaving him but was, against my will, being taken away from him by other forces and agencies over which I had neither control nor interest. It was bull, I had to admit. Maybe not a hundred percent pure, but bull nonetheless.

While my failure brought up useful material in Quentin's last week, I hadn't done him any favor. He'd had plenty to talk about and suffer without my adding insult to his injury. However, it did promote our talking even plainer and better. My taking ownership of my going away to advance my career and life allowed Quentin to share more of his anger at me for leaving, as well as to explore what growing up means, not just pessimistically but optimistically. Most of all, it reinvigorated the trusting relationship we'd both come to rely on. After that consequential hour, Quentin knew that when I said he'd taught me much, I meant it.

These forced terminations carry certain limitations and responsibilities. If the time constraints are known—as they are for a practicum student, intern, or fellow in training—the children and their parents who enter into these relationships deserve to know what they are getting into at the therapy's outset. Beyond the usual tasks (discussed below), these terminations need to involve an added appreciation for cases in which the child requires more therapy, when she hasn't finished her work even though her therapist is leaving.

> "I'm never doing therapy again." Twelve-year-old Tabitha, who perpetually drew pictures, covered her drawing so I couldn't see it.
>
> "But there'll be other therapists you might like even more," I sophomorically suggested.
>
> "I never liked you, so that won't be very hard," Tabitha replied, smiling at her clever jab despite her hurt.

I, a graduate student at that time, recounted the session for my supervisor, who'd overseen my work with this girl for the past eight months. He knew the situation well. He recognized how much of an achievement was the warm connection that Tabitha, a profoundly neglected child, and I shared. Immediately, he gave me credit for trying to do something decent, helping Tabitha give another therapist a try so that she might proceed with the work that was undone.

But his more patient ear heard and taught me otherwise. "Why," he asked, "are you rushing to send her off?" Hurt by what felt like an awful accusation, I began to protest my affection for her and my upset that she had to move on to someone else. He cut me off, though, questioning neither my intentions nor my caring. "You feel so bad for abandoning her that you can't bear to hear her hurt or see her bereft and alone. You want to find her a new parent so as not to feel so rotten about leaving her."

Renewed by this insight, I was able to allow Tabitha most of our remaining few weeks together to process our terminating, which meant for her to get upset, complain, reject me, reject herself, and fall helpless and hopeless at my feet. Contrary to my earlier strategy, I brought up nothing about the promise of a second therapist or a future therapy. We instead wallowed in her present realization that I was leaving her stone-cold in a time of need.

Midway through her next-to-last session and to my astonishment, Tabitha casually mentioned that she wouldn't mind having a woman therapist next time around. This led to our comfortably discussing, in the final hour, Tabitha's spontaneous request that I help find her a new "girl" therapist who, she hoped, would be even better than me. I did. They hit it off, and the treatment relationship worked out splendidly.

In other cases, I've worked with (and supervised students who worked with) children and parents don't want to start again, at least not so fast. For some children, the injury and loss is too great. Anticipating a new therapy and its burdens—getting to know each other, getting to trust each other, having to explain what feels like everything all over again—looms too large and not worth the effort. Understandably, how hard must it be for a child who's deep in the midst of losing her therapist to look enthusiastically to meeting a new one who likewise may leave someday. To lay a guilt trip or overly stress the risks of not resuming treatment can instill resentment that may deter the family's ever coming back for help. For these children and parents, our job is to let them leave with a good feeling for the specific work they have done and for the mental health profession in general, keeping the door open, so to speak.

Fortunately, as we progress in our careers, we get to see more treatments to completion. No longer relying on other agencies or forces to set the end limits of our therapies, we must assess for ourselves, along with the child and her parents, when she has done the work. What are the general indicators that tell us a child may be ready to end her therapy?

Symptoms, such as anxiety or depression, that have vanished or been reduced to tolerable levels. Problematic behaviors that have diminished or disappeared or been replaced by more adaptive and constructive ones. Greater capacities for bearing stress or negative emotions, such as sadness. Grieving that has gone its way. Developmentally stuck phases that have been surpassed. Trauma that has been mastered. Broader areas of functioning that are free from conflict. Improved reality testing and better judgment. Kinder consciences, lessened guilt, and a greater capacity to soothe oneself. Tolerance for ambivalence. Less ambivalence. More confidence and more resiliency. Less narcissistic vulnerability. Better relationships with family and friends. Improved capacities to play, work (mostly in school), and love. More trust and less mistrust. Greater self-control, less inhibition, and more expansive self-expression. Less distractibility. More openness to learning. Fewer headaches or other bodily stresses. Coming to terms with a limitation, such as a learning disability, and growing able and willing to use coping strategies and take constructive assistance that can help compensate. More independence. More dependence. Better separation. More attachment. Assertiveness. Compliance. A capacity to take pride and joy in accomplishments and life. We may define changes in terms of fancy psychological concepts of substance: ego functioning, object relatedness, mastery of impulses, and evolution of self. Or we may more vividly notice a tense body that is relaxed, a sullen face that now smiles.

This abbreviated list of possible criteria speaks mostly to the wide range of issues for which children are brought to therapy. Which ones apply to a particular patient obviously involves our, the child's, and her parents' judgment. Although we may think most of the child growing braver and no longer susceptible to pervasive anguish, her parents may feel that her being able to function at school and home is the greatest mark of success. Our own capacity to see the child in her fullest glory in the context of both her therapy and the facts of her life (i.e., how she is doing on the outside) will make our assessment a doable thing, even if it involves some negotiating among the three players that matter—child, parent, and therapist. Because we see the child each week, we also can be a bit blind to her growth. Occasionally taking a step back and contemplating these criteria, especially in relation to the child's therapeutic goals, can help us to keep track of the therapy's course, of where it's going and where it might end.

While some children may feel sad and insecure about leaving therapy, a majority welcome the news of their readiness to do so as a sign of their success, of their having grown and being given the official sticker attesting to their psychic well-being, health, and strength. Although a therapy hour doesn't take up much of a child's week, children frequently feel as if their schedule is being enormously freed up. "I'll have so much more time to play, hang out, do nothing . . . " their comments may convey.

As a rule, parents no less generally welcome the therapist's judgment that termination is appropriate. However much they support and appreciate our work with their child, being told that their child is in better shape can feel wonderful. That their busy schedules will be relieved of an hour or two just adds icing to the cake, as maybe does the fact that our monthly bills won't come anymore. Parents may wonder whether this is too good to be true, harboring loving apprehension that their child's suffering or bad behaviors will return. But all in all, the decision to terminate a therapy that has come successfully to a natural conclusion is received with optimism and satisfaction.

Once all agree that terminating makes sense—because so much has been accomplished or because of diminishing returns—the issue of timing is faced. For children who've remained somewhat detached from therapy or who continue to have great difficulty knowing what they think and feel, children who use therapy less in terms of the relationship and more to practically solve problems in their lives, I sometimes agree with the parents' suggestion to phase therapy out slowly and less intensely, going to biweekly meetings and then perhaps monthly sessions for a short while. These children will not, I know, make good psychological use of saying good-bye. They need something different; they need to know that I am still there for support. In the way that a child likes to know his mother is there just in case, these children want to know that I am not disappearing. Their termination is more of a "see you for now" (until they decide they wish to see me).

In pacing a termination, I tend to ask for at least a week for every three months of therapy, with a minimum (when possible) of six weeks for even a single year's work. A little longer is always better because it just gives us that much more time to work. For children who've attached firmly to me and the treatment and who can process their experiences with some agility, I suggest keeping the same weekly schedule right to the end. The sameness of routine—in terms of time and frequency—maintains the momentum that has carried the therapy up to that time. To ease up on the schedule risks deflating the therapeutic tension, surrendering the value of the concluding work. Letting up can also give the wrong impression that we are deinvesting in the child, giving her permission to do the same.

> Pam looked a bit puzzled. We'd been discussing her irritation with a friend who had treated her with a superior air.
> "What is it?" I asked.
> "Aren't we supposed to begin ending today?" she asked.
> "We have been," I replied.
> "But," she looked around the office, "everything's the same. Same time. Same office. Same toys. Same you. Same me. You mean we do the same old thing right to the end?"
> I nodded that indeed that was exactly what we would be doing.
> "Good," she replied. "I was afraid I was doing something wrong."

While termination can do more, as we will discuss, the bottom line of a good ending is to continue to provide the basic ingredients—empathy, keen listening, structure, boundaries, presence, confronting, and so on—allowing for the child's continued therapy as it is. Just because we're stopping doesn't mean that's the only subject we discuss. On the contrary, keeping the same steady therapeutic ax to the grindstone, in addition to offering children more time for productive work on their issues, helps them discover that their self-examination has been to a large degree a self-directed process. Proceeding with their therapy under the stress of our impending separation demonstrates to children that they can do the self-analysis and problem solving of therapy by themselves or with others as they go out on their own and for the rest of their lives.

Of course, the burden of working even as they anticipate our stopping is an essential one. Aware of the upcoming loss, children can grow apathetic or discouraged about their lives, fearful that they can't make it alone or simply feeling as if the meaning of their life and its efforts will vanish.

Marcus had made impressive strides in his hard-fought treatment. Hanging on the edge of delinquency, he had become a good student, good athlete, class leader, responsible friend, loyal son, and reliable patient. The determination to terminate his therapy had exhilarated him. He realized how far he'd come, and he much appreciated his parents' and my vote of confidence in his growth.

Marcus began the termination process apparently pleased and looking forward to being done with treatment. With a few weeks to go, however, his life began to fall apart. He got detentions in school for coming late and unprepared to class, then got detentions on detentions for not showing up for those after-school punishments. At home he verbally assaulted his parents when they confronted his problems at school and threw tantrums when almost anything didn't go as he wished. He skipped basketball practice and began to smoke cigarettes, something he hadn't done for over two years.

Neither his parents nor the school were terribly thrown by this backslide. I'd warned them of the possibility at the time we'd decided on terminating. But Marcus was. "See?" he said. "The therapy didn't work. You were wrong, I'm in worse shape than when I came."

I smiled to myself, recalling the boy who, then truly at great risk, had first come to me. That boy took over a year before he'd been able to acknowledge that his life was anything less than perfect.

"I'm not ready to stop therapy. I'm at risk," he continued.

"At risk for what?" I asked, reassured and not troubled by what I was hearing. Children at real risk tend not to discuss their risk in this manner, nor do they as a rule want or think they need the help of therapy.

"I don't know," Marcus said, tripped by my actually asking. "Everything."

I looked Marcus in the eye. "There's only one thing you're at risk for, and it's not failing school, or getting into trouble, or using drugs, or any of the other stuff you've mentioned. And I think you know what that is."

"What is it?" Marcus asked, having lost the bluster of his argument, appearing to both want and not want the answer.

"Missing me."

Several minutes of silence passed before Marcus spoke. "It seems kind of unfair that just when you're doing really good, you lose the thing that helped you get there."

"You're right," I agreed. "It is unfair."

His not-so-unconscious wish to prove that he still needed me and therapy having been brought to the light of day, Marcus instantaneously regrouped and left therapy walking tall and straight.

Under the stress of termination, symptoms and old behaviors commonly return or intensify. They can be in the service of soliciting the therapist's help and concern (as were Marcus's), or they can have other, infinitely varied and unique meanings related to the child's previous ways of coping with loss. In a therapy that has proceeded well and coherently, these temporary regressions need not overly worry us.

For months, actually since we began, Seth had pleaded not to have to come to treatment. He originally came with a myriad of symptoms that included stomachaches, high anxiety, school phobia, inhibition, skin rashes that broke out under stress, and constant irritability—most of which had subsided dramatically. Now his wish was coming true; he could really quit.

Like Marcus, Seth was elated. "Now I can play with friends," he speculated. "And watch television. And work on my go-cart. Bike ride, roller blade, swim, and skate. And just hang out, too." Seth had what sounded to be hundreds of hours of new activity slated to fill in the one free hour a week he was gaining (a sign, I hadn't yet realized, of the enormous void he was anticipating).

But a couple of weeks following our joint decision to terminate, Seth grew more anxious. He had to leave school because of nausea and stomach pains and resisted going back. He grew clingy and refused to leave his mother for a dentist's appointment and a soccer practice. A friend's birthday party panicked him enough to stay home. Most obvious of all, he broke out in hives over most of his body.

Seth's regression disturbed his parents. Their fear (a near universal one for child patients and their parents) that his gains had been transitory or even illusory appeared to be coming true. "Maybe he shouldn't stop," they wondered aloud. "Maybe therapy's never worked, or maybe he needs it forever," they added, the ambivalence of their doubt so wonderfully expressed in these polar opposites. "Can't you do something?"

I completely appreciated their distress. But I knew what had to be done. Knowing that we'd made the determination to end therapy thoughtfully and slowly and that it was a good decision, I reminded myself of the need to stay steady in the wake of this regression.

"Send Seth to school," I recommended matter-of-factly. "Don't pamper or medicate his bodily complaints. And he doesn't need to see a doctor." For he'd been evaluated thoroughly for all of his symptoms. "Basically, keep doing all of the good things you've learned to do over the past years of our work together."

"You mean the structure and the limits?" his mother asked. "But he seems so vulnerable right now."

I agreed that he was, stressing that the same reliable consistency was needed now, perhaps more than ever.

Likewise, I fended off my temptation to coddle Seth in a way I never had. Feeling bad that he would no longer have me, I felt a need to be more available, more active, more helpful, more supportive, more reassuring, more of everything. After all, in a short few weeks he wouldn't have me at all. But I knew better. To try and pour years of me into a handful of sessions might have alleviated my needs, but it would have harshly ignored and prolonged Seth's. Like a mother who feels guilt-ridden about her soon-to-be-born second child, who seductively invites her first child to regress, to be more of the baby, I would be setting Seth up for a certain fall if I gave him more and more just as I was about to be there not at all.

Enlightened by this self-counseling, I held back, making space for Seth to fend more for himself. "You're not helping me!" he exclaimed. "You're no good anymore," he became convinced. "I don't even know why I ever liked you."

Under my watchful if reserved eye, Seth floundered in his misery until ultimately, through his tears and gasps, he expressed his rage that I would be leaving him. I didn't mention that it was actually he who would be leaving me; that was irrelevant for now. Seth had it right. He would have to manage much of his hurt, and pleasure, and life, by himself.

Just as we had judged, Seth was indeed ready and capable of doing so. His cascade of old troubles came and went, a last hurrah for his more infantile means of coping that, however maladaptive and painful, had been precious to him. To give up old symptoms and behaviors meant to give up what was before, to put the past where it belonged—in the past.

Those regressions of termination, as well the more conscious reflecting that takes place, can allow for a remembering of what has gone before. In these final hours, children will recall the states in which they began therapy, often pondering where they would have been had it not been for therapy and reviewing their gains. They may pine nostalgically for what was, as well as look forward to the growth and life that lies ahead. Occasionally a child will make a book of therapy memories or some other concrete creation by which to document our time together. More commonly, children will find themselves, perhaps quite unknowingly, revisiting old games, old activities, and old play that we shared, especially early on in the therapy.

Of course, the mother of all issues that terminating evokes is the obvious: the child's leaving of us and all that we've supplied—our holding, accepting, admiring, interest, patience, and belief that she holds the key, potential, and responsibility to overcome and grow.

Sara wanted to be a good girl, but she notoriously gave people a different impression. She was a child whose energy level could rival that of any nuclear particle, whose best intentions always seemed to go astray. Distractible and quite active, she was ever unwittingly creating mishaps with her fidgeting hands and feet, body parts that constantly sought stimulation, boundaries, and contact with others. Her constant questions and requests, then demands, for attention drained her much quieter, reserved parents.

Her complexity of personality and ego made her no less curious and challenging in school. A very bright child who could also act dumb when she chose, Sara worked hard for and was loved by some teachers. She could do little—or less—for other teachers, who came close to disdaining her. A magnetic personality who tended to attract or repel others, Sara left few people feeling indifferent toward her. When she had entered therapy, she was being followed closely by an eminent child psychiatrist and was on a medication that her parents judged to be helping with her concentration and impulsivity.

Yet both the parents and the psychiatrist felt there was more to her story. Psychological testing conducted before meeting me showed a proneness to depression, low self-esteem, lack of confidence in her ability to manage herself, and an exquisite vulnerability to narcissistic injury.

From our initial handshake, Sara and I became fast allies in her self-exploration. Unfortunately, the task was to be much more arduous and trying than Sara anticipated. For months Sara would come to me, complaining of the gross mistreatment that she felt much of the world gave her. Once secure in the therapeutic environment distinguished by patience, empathy, and nonintrusion, Sara talked with increasing openness about the barbs and arrows of life that seemed to lodge in her skin. For the first time in her life, her parents reported, she could admit to the unhappiness that others could see in her. That she might be contributing to any of her difficulties, however, was not a remote consideration.

When Sara and I butted heads (which wasn't often, for I was one of the good guys she worked hard to please), she tried to sidestep the issue, upping her attempt to charm and distract me. But one day, many months into treatment, Sara couldn't find enough space to run around a problem we shared. Cleaning up the office by wildly throwing toys backwards over her head at the toy box, she hit a framed picture with a small wooden block. We both knew what the cracking sound was before we even checked.

"I didn't mean it. Really, I didn't. I'm sorry. I'll pay for it." Sara apologized a mile a minute. "I wasn't trying to break the glass. I swear I wasn't."

I stayed silent, allowing Sara to flail.

"I don't know what gets into me," she bemoaned aloud. "I'm always screwing up. No matter what I try to do, it turns out bad. I tried to make my dad a gift for Father's Day, and I ended up getting glue all over his desk. He was furious and told me he'd rather I didn't make him gifts." Talking at the speed of light, Sara poured out her long-aching heart of the many assorted ways she'd made a mess of things. In between each avalanche of revelation, she'd cry and cry.

That momentous occasion led to Sara's being able to examine, therapeutic molecule by molecule, the erratic and troubling incidents that pervaded her life. "Mrs. Collins hates me," she'd say, only to follow my empathic understanding for how bad that must feel with admissions as to what she'd done to get the teacher's goat. In her tedious and tortuous reconstruction, Sara began making distinctions between the *can't* and the *won't* of her trials and tribulations. Acknowledging more the frustration for times when she couldn't control herself and her actions led her to recognize the more-numerous-than-she'd-reckoned times when she could. Gaining the capacity to slow herself down, to contemplate and analyze the things she would do and what would happen to her as a result, brought insights into unconscious motivations for some of her action.

"My father thinks it's my ADD that makes me kick the back of his car seat," she decided. "But I really want to annoy him 'cause he thinks my sister's so much better." She similarly deciphered her not passing in homework she'd done ("No one's going to tell me what to do or when to do it") and her insulting of peers ("They all think they're so much better than I am") as well as many other facets of her attitude and behavior. While seeing more of the thoughts and feelings that went into her difficulties, she also came to better terms with her neurological susceptibility to distractibility and impulsivity. "I wish I was calm like a lake," she sighed.

Her work progressed much further than any of us would have predicted, and the day came when Sara and her parents broached the question of termination. With apparent glee, Sara looked at my calendar, deciding, with my approval, that we should meet for eight more weeks.

Sara used that time well. She kept on analyzing the little pieces of life that pricked her skin and threatened her much stabilized ego. She actively worked on developing strategies to help her help herself, extrapolating the functions of myself to herself. For example, she decided that she could listen to herself carefully, just as I would do, before criticizing herself for something that went wrong. But in spite of all this able and worthy work that prepared for her terminating, Sara, in the first seven of our remaining eight hours, made no direct mention of our coming end.

It was not until the final hour that Sara made those sentiments known more fully. She had walked into the office behind my back while I was sitting at my desk.

"I'm sorry," I began to speak while putting my pencil down and closing up my scheduling book, "I was just writing . . . " Sara burst into tears.

"What is it, Sara?" I queried, knowing she was sad about our ending but not knowing what specifically had precipitated her distress. She pointed to my appointment book.

"This?" I asked.

"Someone," she began to speak, but her emotions choked her. Minutes later, she explained. "Someone else is coming to see you next week." Again she broke down. "We're really stopping, aren't we?"

"Yes, we are, Sara. We are."

The feelings that had propelled the fine work she'd been able to do throughout the termination phase were held in this small packet and could wait no longer to be freed. The end had come.

Termination, in its fullest and richest sense, awakens children's deepest fears of separation, loss, and abandonment. For some, termination can resemble a psychic approximation of death, giving the anguishing impression that they are losing someone most dear to them—forever. It is a metaphor for the good-bye of good-byes; children confront the longings that they most cherish. In their hard work they have come to more realistic terms with who they and their loved ones are. They have likely surrendered unreachable ideals that have haunted and punished them for being less. Putting some of their past in its proper place, they have grieved people, places, and things. Odd or trite as it may sound, they have even grieved for the selves they once fancied they could be and for the children they never will be again. And besides just giving up their longings for and fantasies of the therapists they imagined we might be, they must give up the real therapists who saw them through it all.

From their very first step into our office, we have worked ever hard to make children's contact with us a worthwhile one. For some children the play and talk of therapy comes easily and with pleasure, our presence a constant comfort and support. For others the kinship is much rougher, that same play and talk an onerous burden and source of humiliation and resentment. Whatever the course of our relationship and however successful or frustrating the outcome, we strive to send children out from therapy able to take pride and joy in a job well done and on footing surer than they came in on, with the promise of sustained growth and continuing progress as they return to a life without us.

References

Abbott, K. (1990). The use of play in the psychological preparation of preschool children undergoing cardiac surgery. *Issues in Comprehensive Pediatric Nursing, 13,* 265–277.

Ack, M., Beale, E., & Ware, L. (1975). Parent guidance: Psychotherapy of the young child via the parent. *Bulletin of the Menninger Clinic, 39*(5), 436–447.

Allen, F. H. (1964). The beginning phase of therapy. In M. R. Haworth (Ed.), *Child psychotherapy* (pp. 101–105). New York: Basic Books.

American Psychiatric Association. (2000). *Diagnostic and statistical manual of mental disorders* (4th ed.).Washington, DC: Author.

Arnold, E. (1978). *Helping parents help their children.* New York: Brunner/ Mezel.

Axline, V. M. (1947). *Play therapy.* Boston: Houghton Mifflin.

Axline, V. M. (1964). *Dibs: In search of self.* Boston: Houghton Mifflin.

Baggs, A. M. (2000). The validity of autistic opinions. *Autistic Information Library.* www.autistics.org/library/autopin.html.

Basch, M. (1995). *Doing brief treatment.* New York: Basic Books.

Bellinson, J. (2002). *Children's use of board games in psychotherapy.* Northvale, NJ: Aronson.

Berke, J. H., Navaratnem, K., & Schonfield, T. (2006). Creative use of the countertransference. *British Journal of Psychotherapy, 22,* 311–328.

Bostic J. Q. (2001). Psychiatric school consultation: An organizing framework and empowering techniques. *Child and Adolescent Psychiatric Clinics of North America, 10,* 1–12.

Bromfield, R. (1989). Psychodynamic play therapy with a high-functioning autistic child. *Psychoanalytic Psychology, 6,* 439–453.

Bromfield, R. (1992). *Playing for real.* New York: Dutton.

Bromfield, R. (1995). The use of puppets in play therapy. *Child and Adolescent Social Work Journal, 12,* 435–444.

Bromfield, R. (1996). Yes (Point/Counterpoint). *Priorities, 3,* 24–26.

Bromfield, R. (2000). It's the tortoise's race: Long-term psychodynamic therapy with a high-functioning autistic adolescent. *Psychoanalytic Inquiry, 20,* 732–745.

Bromfield, R. (2005). *Teens in therapy: Making it their own.* New York: Norton.

Bromfield, R. (2006). *Playing for real: Exploring the world of play therapy and the inner worlds of children* (Rev. ed.). Hamilton, MA: BasilBooks .com.

Bromfield, R. & Erwin, C. (2001). *How to turn boys into men without a man around the house.* Roseville, CA: Prima.

Chethik, M. (1976). Work with parents: Treatment of the parent-child relationship. *Journal of the American Academy of Child and Adolescent Psychiatry, 15,* 453–463.

Colm, H. (1964). A field theory approach to transference and its particular application to children. In M. Haworth (Ed.), *Child psychotherapy* (pp. 242–256). New York: Basic Books.

Corwin, M. D. (2001). *Brief treatment in clinical social work practice.* Pacific Grove, CA: Wadsworth.

Cosgrove, L., & Krimsky, S. (2006). Financial ties between DSM-IV panel members and the pharmaceutical industry. *Psychotherapy and Psychosomatics, 75,* 154–160.

Dawley, A. (1939). Interrelated movement of parent and child in therapy with children. *American Journal of Orthopsychiatry, 9*(4), 748–754.

Ekstein, R. (1966). *Children of time and space of action and impulse.* New York: Aronson.

Ekstein, R., & Wallerstein, J. (1956). Observations on the psychotherapy of borderline and psychotic children. *Psychoanalytic Study of the Child, 11,* 303–311.

Ekstein, R., Wallerstein, J. S., & Mandelbaum, A. (1992). Countertransference in the residential treatment of children. In J. R. Brandell

(Ed.), *Countertransference in psychotherapy with children and adolescents* (pp. 59–87). Lanham, MD: Aronson.

Freud, A. (1927). The role of transference in the analysis of children. In *The Writings of Anna Freud* (Vol. 1, pp. 36–49). New York: International Universities Press.

Freud, A. (1928). Introduction to the techniques of child analysis. *Nervous and Mental Disease Monograph, 28.*

Gardner, R. (1990). *Psychotherapeutic approaches to the resistant child.* Northvale, NJ: Aronson.

Gil, E., & Drewes, A. A. (2005). *Cultural issues in play therapy.* New York: Guilford.

Ginott, H. (1959). The theory and practice of therapeutic intervention in child treatment. *Journal of Consulting Psychology, 23,* 160–166.

Ginott, H. (1961). *Group psychotherapy with children.* New York: McGraw-Hill.

Ginott, H. (1968). Interpretations and child therapy. In E. Hammer (Ed.), *Use of interpretation in treatment* (pp. 291–294). New York: Grune and Stratton.

Greenberg, J. R., & Mitchell, S. A. (1983). *Object relations in psychoanalytic theory.* Cambridge, MA: Harvard University Press.

Hall, K. (2000). *Asperger syndrome, the universe, and everything.* London: Jessica Kingsley.

Harris, A. (2004). The experience of silence: A client case study. *Counseling Psychology Review, 19,* 5–11.

Haworth, M. R. (1964). *Child psychotherapy: Practice and theory.* New York: Basic Books.

Hoffman, D. L., & Remmel, M. L. (1975). Uncovering the precipitant in crisis intervention. *Social Casework, 56,* 259–267.

Kaduson, H., & Schaefer, C. (1997). *101 play therapy techniques.* Northvale, NJ: Aronson.

Kaduson, H., & Schaefer, C. (2000a). *101 more play therapy techniques* (Vol. 2). Northvale, NJ: Aronson.

Kaduson, H., & Schaefer, C. (2000b). *Short-term play therapy for children.* Northvale, NJ: Aronson.

Kaduson, H., & Schaefer, C. (2003). *101 more play therapy techniques* (Vol. 3). Northvale, NJ: Aronson.

Kendall, J. (2003, February 9). Managed care tried to kill off Freud: Can Tony Soprano help revive him. *Boston Globe,* p. D1.

King, P., & Steiner, R. (1991). *The Freud-Klein controversies 1941–45.* London: Routledge.

Klein, M. (1932). *The psychoanalysis of children.* London: Hogarth.

Klorer, P. G. (2000). *Expressive therapy with troubled children.* Northvale, NJ: Aronson.

Kohut, H. (1977). *The restoration of the self*. New York: International Universities Press.

Kohut, H. (1987). *The Kohut seminars on self psychology and psychotherapy with adolescents and young adults*. New York: Norton.

Lanyado, M. (2004). *The presence of the therapist: Treating childhood trauma*. New York: Brunner Routledge.

Lawrence-Lightfoot, S. K. (2003). *The essential conversation*. New York: Ballantine.

Linn, S. (1986). Puppet therapy with pediatric bone marrow transplant patients. *Journal of Pediatric Psychology, 11*, 37–46.

Malawista, K. L. (2004). Rescue fantasies in child therapy: Countertransference/transference enactments. *Child and Adolescent Social Work Journal, 21*, 373–386.

Malchiodi, C. (1997). *Breaking the silence: Art therapy with children from violent homes*. New York: Brunner/Mazel.

Malchiodi, C. (1998). *Understanding children's drawings*. New York: Guilford.

Masterson, J. F. (1972). *Treatment of the borderline adolescent: A developmental approach*. New York: Wiley-Interscience.

Meeks, J. E., & Bernet, W. (2001). *The fragile alliance*. Melbourne, FL: Krieger.

Merriam-Webster's collegiate dictionary (10th ed.). (1993). Springfield, MA: Merriam-Webster.

Miller, J. P. (1996). *Using self psychology in child psychotherapy: The restoration of the child*. Northvale, NJ: Aronson.

Moustakas, C. (1959). *Psychotherapy with children*. New York: Harper & Row.

Nagelberg, L., & Feldman, Y. (1953). The attempt at healthy insulation in the withdrawn child. *American Journal of Orthopsychiatry, 3*, 238–251.

Novick, K., & Novick, J. (2005). *Working with parents makes therapy work*. Northvale, NJ: Aronson.

Oberschneider, M. S. (2002). Understanding transference in parent guidance. *Bulletin of the Menninger Clinic, 66*, 184–205.

Pine, F. (1974). On the concept "borderline" in children. *Psychoanalytic Study of the Child, 29*, 341–368.

Pine, F. (1988). The four psychologies of psychoanalysis and their place in clinical work. *Journal of the American Psychoanalytic Association, 36*, 571–596.

Prado de Oliveira, L. E. (2001). The nature of the transference between Anna Freud and Melanie Klein. *International Forum of Psychoanalysis, 10*, 247–258.

Rambert, M. (1949). *Children in conflict*. New York: International Universities Press.

Reisman, J. M. (1973). *Principles of psychotherapy with children.* New York: Wiley.

Riley, S. (1999). *Contemporary art therapy with adolescents.* London: Jessica Kingsley.

Rogers, C. (1951). *Client-centered therapy.* Boston: Houghton Mifflin.

Rubin, J. A. (2005). *Child art therapy.* Hoboken, NJ: Wiley.

Sandler, J., Kennedy, H., & Tyson, R. L. (Eds.). (1980). *The technique of child psychoanalysis: Discussions with Anna Freud.* Cambridge, MA: Harvard University Press.

Schaefer, C. (2003). *Foundations of play therapy.* Hoboken, NJ: Wiley.

Schaefer, C., & Cangelosi, D. (Eds.). (2002). *Play therapy techniques* (2nd ed.). Lanham, MD: Aronson.

Schaefer, C., & Reid, S. E. (2001). *Game play: Therapeutic use of childhood games.* Hoboken, NJ: Wiley.

Schroder, D. (2004). *Little windows into art therapy: Small openings for beginning therapists.* London: Jessica Kingsley.

Segal, H. (1964). *Introduction to the work of Melanie Klein.* London: Hogarth.

Seinfield, J. (1993). *Interpreting and holding: The paternal and maternal functions of the psychotherapist.* Northvale, NJ: Aronson.

Selekman, M. D. (2002). *Living on the razor's edge: Solution-oriented brief family therapy with self-harming adolescents.* New York: Norton.

Shapiro, J. P., Friedberg, R. D., & Bardenstein, K. K. (2006). *Child and adolescent therapy: Science and art.* Hoboken, NJ: Wiley.

Sifneos, P. (2004). *Short-term psychodynamic psychotherapy, evaluation, and technique.* New York: Springer.

Silverman, D. K. (2006). What works in psychotherapy and how do we know? What evidence-based practice has to offer. *Psychoanalytic Psychology, 22,* 306–312.

Siskind, D. (1997). *Working with parents.* Northvale, NJ: Aronson.

Sperling, M. (1994). *The major neuroses and behavior disorders in children.* Northvale, NJ: Jason Aronson.

Storr, A. (1988). *Solitude: A return to the self.* New York: Free Press.

Sutton, A. (1991). Deprivation entangled and disentangled. *Journal of Child Psychotherapy, 17,* 61–77.

Terr, L. C. (2003). Wild child: How three principles of healing organized 12 years of psychotherapy. *Journal of the American Academy of Child and Adolescent Psychiatry, 42,* 1401–1409.

Terr, L. C. (2006). When formulation outweighs diagnosis: 13 "moments" in psychotherapy. *Journal of the American Academy of Child and Adolescent Psychiatry, 45,* 1252–1263.

Terr, L. C., et al. (2005). Moments in psychotherapy. *Journal of the American Academy of Child and Adolescent Psychiatry, 44,* 191–197.

Tolpin, M. (1971). On the beginnings of a cohesive self. *The Psychoanalytic Study of the Child, 26,* 316–352.

Varon, L. (2000). *Adopting on your own.* New York: Farrar, Straus and Giroux.

Weisz, J. R. (2004). *Psychotherapy for children and adolescents.* New York: Cambridge University Press.

Winnicott, D. (1974). *Playing and reality.* New York: Penguin.

Winnicott, D. (1975a). Primitive emotional development. In D. Winnicott (Ed.), *Through pediatrics to psycho-analysis* (pp. 145–156). New York: Basic.

Winnicott, D. (1975b). Transitional objects and transitional phenomena. In D. Winnicott (Ed.), *Through pediatrics to psycho-analysis* (pp. 229–242). New York: Basic.

Index

A

Abbott, K., 83
Abreaction, 31–32
Abuse, asking about, 18
Abused child, 18, 42, 69, 70,
    78, 86–87, 114, 134,
    138–139
Abusive child, 134, 187–190
Ack, M., 175

Action figures, 84. *See also*
    Puppet play
Admiring the child, 37, 44
Affection, setting limits on,
    58–59, 154–157
Aggression, 36, 133
Aggression in therapy,
    setting limits on, 55–59,
    156–157

Because this is a book about technique, I refrain from debate concerning specific diagnoses. Accordingly, readers will find, for example, that a case involving impulsive behavior may be indexed under "Impulsive child," "Borderline child," "Bipolar child," and "Self-injury." Likewise, material relevant to both Asperger's and high-functioning autism are referenced to each entity. The entry "Narcissistically vulnerable child" includes material related to both the narcissistic child and the child with narcissistic issues. My goal is simply to help clinician readers find what they seek easily and directly.

About the Author

Richard Bromfield, Ph.D., is a graduate of Bowdoin College and the University of North Carolina at Chapel Hill. A faculty member of Harvard Medical School at the Massachusetts Mental Health Center, he writes about children, psychotherapy, and family life in both professional and popular periodicals. He is author of *Playing for Real: Exploring the World of Play Therapy and the Inner Worlds of Children, Teens in Therapy: Making It Their Own, Handle with Care: Understanding Children and Teachers,* and several books for parents. Dr. Bromfield has a private practice with children and adults in both Boston and Danvers, Massachusetts.